Leadership Skills for Licensed Practical Nurses Working with the Aging Population

Cheryl Kruschke

Leadership Skills for Licensed Practical Nurses Working with the Aging Population

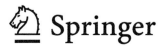 Springer

Cheryl Kruschke
Loretto Heights School of Nursing
Regis University
Denver, Colorado
USA

ISBN 978-3-030-09918-3   ISBN 978-3-319-69862-5   (eBook)
https://doi.org/10.1007/978-3-319-69862-5

Printed on acid-free paper

This Springer imprint is published by Springer Nature
The registered company is Springer International Publishing AG
The registered company address is: Gewerbestrasse 11, 6330 Cham, Switzerland

I dedicate this book to my husband Robert; you have remained at my side for 38 years, helping me reach my dreams among the stars.
To my children Michelle and Joe (Kelly) and our Angel Jeffrey; grandchildren Katie (Chris), Nikki, Kyle, Jonny, Lily, and Emma; and great-grandchild Theodore.
Your love means more than words can express.
To my sister Deb for your help with this book.

Contents

Introduction

1

In this chapter, you will review the history of our health-care system and nursing homes, the history of nursing and the licensed practical nurse, and the current trends in nursing including my journey to write this book. Through this book you will be able to fill gaps in your own practice related to leadership, management, culture change, and person-directed care concepts. Let's look back before we move forward.

1.1 History of US Health-Care System and Nursing Homes

Providing care to each other has historical connotations that date back as far as we can surmise. Initially, care was provided by immediate family members. The first "professional" caregivers were those individuals interested in the art of healing based on variety of premises including religious beliefs or folk healing beliefs. We are all familiar with the red and white striped barber pole that has come to represent a location where our hair can be cut. Initially, barbers could also be caregivers/surgeons. This also applies to religious leaders as well as dentists.

Eventually, the need to be professionally trained as a physician resulted in the establishment of the American Medical Association in 1847. Through the efforts of this organization, the role of the physician became truly professional based on a higher level of education at the university level. During the same time period, health care began to move away from the private home. Poor houses were established to provide care to those who were unable to pay. Hospitals were set up to provide a practice location for physicians and to establish care environments that reached a wider population beyond indigent individuals (Niles 2014). Initially, most hospitals were owned by physicians. Eventually government entities developed hospitals to ensure indigent populations received appropriate care. Hospitals with religious affiliations were formed, and higher education organizations developed hospitals as a base for the education of physicians and eventually nurses.

© Springer International Publishing AG 2018   1
C. Kruschke, *Leadership Skills for Licensed Practical Nurses Working
with the Aging Population*, https://doi.org/10.1007/978-3-319-69862-5_1

In 1965, President Johnson signed the law initiating Medicare and Medicaid programs. This legislation provided the catalyst for the proliferation of nursing homes through government funding. Traditional long-term care settings were developed based on the medical model of nursing that reflected the hospital setting (Kruschke 2006; Ragsdale and McDougall 2008). Consumers are no longer willing to accept this model of care for older populations. As our population of aging individuals continue to grow, the problem of how nursing homes function will become even more pronounced, and the need for caregiving will become even more focused. The aging population of the United States reflect what is happening across the globe. The population of individuals over the age of 65 in the United States was approximately 46.2 million in 2014 (Administration on Aging 2016). There are 15,600 nursing homes in the United States with 1.7 million nursing home beds and 1,340,700 residents representing an average occupancy rate of 79% (Centers for Disease Control and Prevention 2016). According to the Department of Health and Human Services, Administration on Aging (2016), the US population of older persons will continue to grow exponentially between 2010 and 2040 as we experience the aging of the "baby boomer" generation. It is anticipated the population of individuals over the age of 65 will increase to 21.7% of the overall population in the United States (para. 1). This represents a significant increase that cannot be ignored. "Demand for long-term care will increase significantly when baby boomers with declining health demand more individualized activities and services. Expenditures for nursing home care are expected to exceed $100 billion annually by the year 2050" (Deutschman 2005, p. 247).

1.2   History of Nursing

Understanding the role of the licensed practical nurse (LPN) or licensed vocational nurse (LVN) requires us to look back at the history of caregiving. Caregivers were members of the immediate family and extended family members. This role tended to be female including the wife, grandmothers, aunts, and adult daughters. It was not uncommon for female members of the family to be called to the bedside of relatives to tend them during illness, birth of a child, injury, and even at the time of death.

During war, women were also called upon to tend the injured. While the care they were able to provide was basic, they learned techniques to provide care through older family members, physicians if available, and "nurses." These women were specially trained by physicians to provide first aid. They assisted the physician in the care of the ill and injured. Eventually, nursing programs were developed to formalize the training of women as nurses. The first training programs were based on the teachings of Florence Nightingale who was the founder of modern nursing. Through her work during the Crimean War, nursing techniques that embrace the entire person were developed and advocated. When she returned from the war, she opened the first professional school of nursing in London, England (Egenes 2009).

When the Civil War broke out in the United States, there were no professional nurses available to care for the soldiers. Women who had cared for their family members volunteered to care for the soldiers. These women were the first official nurses in the United States. Their shared vision for formal education evolved into the first nursing schools to train future nurses. They started their training in alms-houses, which eventually became the first hospitals in the United States. Formal education evolved into schools of nursing attached to the local hospitals, providing women with education, while they provided the bulk of the care to patients in those hospitals. Student nurses often lived near the ward they worked on, and training occurred in classrooms nearby as well. These nursing programs became the precursor for diploma programs that sprung up across the United States to educate nurses. These programs usually lasted 3 years with on-the-job training as the exemplar.

In the early 1900s, states began developing exams nurses would take to prove proficiency in the field. During World War II, the need for nurses flourished once again. Many nurses became employed through the Civil Works Administration (Nursingdegreeguide.org 2017). It was not until after World War II when licensing became a requirement for nurses graduating from formal programs. After World War II, a nursing shortage developed as women opted to return home and raise families. Due to this shortage, Associate Degree Nursing (ADN) programs were developed to graduate nurses more quickly. The ADN program was very successful at graduating nurses who had the technical skills needed to be proficient at the bedside. These nurses took the same exams as the diploma and degree program nurses, making ADN programs a success. In the mid-1960s the American Nurses Association took the position nursing education should move from the hospital setting to the university setting (Egenes 2009).

1.3   History of the Licensed Practical Nurse

In the acute care setting, having a variety of strategies to staff nursing units helps to overcome the nursing shortage. One staffing strategy is primary care nursing which teams registered nurses (RNs) and unlicensed personnel such as certified nursing assistants (CNAs) providing care as team members. The RN provides nursing care to 4 or 5 patients while the CNA provides hands-on care for the activities of daily living (ADLs) for 10 to 12 patients. One CNA will be teamed with 2 or 3 RNs. The third person that may or may not be used as part of the team approach is the licensed practical nurse (LPN) or licensed vocational nurse (LVN). This member of the team would be assigned to complete treatments and medication administration excluding specific medications only the RN can give. Both the LPN and CNA would work under the direct supervision of the RN.

In the long-term care setting, the RN and the LPN work in similar roles. Both the RN and the LPN can be the lead nurse on a given unit. However, the LPN is not able to perform assessments and cannot start an IV without specific certification. The LPN is able to contact physicians, delegate to CNAs, and perform the functions of a unit nurse similar to the RN. In the home health setting, LPNs are in practice but not to the extent they are used in the nursing home setting.

A report by the Health Resources and Services Administration (2004) acknowledged the role of the licensed practical nurse in the nursing home setting. In many
cases, the role of the LPN is similar to that of the RN with restrictions based on the
licensing body in each state. Regardless, this study also spoke to the importance of
education in improving resident outcomes in the nursing home setting. The
American Health Care Association (2008) indicates that the turnover rate for LPNs
is 60% with one in nine LPN positions being vacant. "The high vacancy rates confirm that there is a continuing need for government policy and educational initiatives to promote careers in long term care nursing. High quality nursing facility
services depend upon a stable, well-trained workforce" (p.i.).

1.4   Current Trends in Nursing

With the aging of the baby boomers, the need for health-care services in the United
States is anticipated to grow. This will bring a rise in cost and the need for new
technologies which will also result in an increase in cost (Li et al. 2017). Using
unlicensed personnel to provide basic hands-on care to patients under the supervision of the registered nurse is not an unusual practice, especially to save money or
to offset nursing shortages. Currently, LPNs are used most often in the long-term
care setting. As reported by Li et al. (2017), the average number of work hours for
LPNs declined 35.5% between 2010 and 2014 in the hospital setting. At the same
time, the RN hours remained stable, and the use of unlicensed assistive personnel,
the CNA, declined by 14.2%, while the graduate nurse increased by 75.4%.

This shift in the use of LPNs in the acute care setting may be driven by associated or perceived patient outcomes and satisfaction linked to the educational level
of the hospital nursing staff including RNs, LPNs, and CNAs. Hockenberry and
Becker (2016), completed a study by collecting data for 3 years from 311
California hospitals. The goal of this study was to determine if and what impact
nursing staff had on patient satisfaction and whether or not patient satisfaction
scores improved when care was provided primarily by RNs. The results indicated
a marginal improvement in satisfaction scores related to higher levels of RNs
staffing the units. However, if LPN/LVN hours were increased, patient satisfaction based on recommending the hospital to others declined. Overall, the skill
level of each nurse was far more important than the level of education alone in
improving satisfaction score. This is only one example of the studies currently
being implemented to research patient outcomes and satisfaction related to skill
level and educational level of licensed nurses. Given the number of studies that
determined skill level and educational level of licensed nurses' impact on patient
outcomes and satisfaction, the proliferation of nursing programs to advance education of entry-level nurses to the degreed level has increased. While the implication is that the degreed nurse is the registered nurse, the National League for
Nursing (NLN) has taken the position that the nursing community needs to work
with LPNs/LVNs to develop an inclusive workforce that "ensures that all nurses

who touch patients daily in varied health care settings are acknowledged as essential partners to meet the varied needs of today's complex health care system" (National League for Nursing 2014, p. 418).

According to the NLN, the growth in employment for LPNs/LVNs is expected to grow by 22% through the year 2020. The NLN also reported that the National Council of State Boards of Nursing (NCSBN) indicated that 54% of LPNs/LVNs work in long-term care settings such as a nursing home, while 25% of LPNs/LVNs work in community-based facilities or programs. Additionally, 70% of licensed nursing care in the nursing home setting is provided by LPNs/LVNs, and 40% of those nurses reported completing administrative duties as well (National League for Nursing 2014). These trends require us to ensure the LPN/LVN receives recognition for the essential role they play as part of the patient care team and to ensure LPNs/LVNs receive advanced education in keeping with their role as a practitioner in health-care settings that reach vulnerable populations such as our aging population. In honor of all LPNs, I made the decision to write this book.

1.5   About the Author

I began my nursing career in 1980 as a licensed practical nurse (LPN). The two hospitals in my community transitioned to primary care nursing while I was in school. When I completed the program, the only job I was able to obtain was working in a nursing home. I often tell people that I began caring for older adults by chance and stayed by choice. I was an LPN for 24 years, during which time I developed and honed my nursing skills in the nursing home setting. I worked in a variety of roles throughout my career as an LPN including a unit nurse, supervisor, MDS coordinator, and even nursing home administrator. I was fortunate that I had gone back to school and obtained a business degree and a master's degree while maintaining my role as a LPN. These programs taught me a great deal regarding management and leadership, which helped me to understand my role as a nurse in the long-term care setting.

After 22 years as a LPN, I decided to return to school and obtain my associate degree in nursing. Right from the start, I realized there were key elements of my education as a registered nurse that were missing from the education I received as an LPN including leadership, management, and communication skills beyond the classroom. Additionally, current trends in health care including culture change and person-directed care have come to the forefront, requiring not only the understanding of these concepts but how to apply them to practice in the clinical setting.

Throughout the registered nurse program, I had multiple "aha moments" that I shared with my peers and my team. I began to formulate an idea for an educational program that would assist LPNs to obtain the missing concepts based on my own experience and the experiences of other LPNs. I continued my education journey, resulting in a bachelor's degree in nursing, a master's degree in nursing, and a doctorate degree in education.

As an educator, I have been honored to work with hundreds of nursing students working to obtain their master's and doctorate degrees in nursing. I never lost sight of my idea for an educational program for LPNs. I obtained a grant to develop this program and implemented it with a group of 15 LPNs based on my experiences working as an LPN.

1.6   Presentation of Concepts

As I indicated previously, while I was attending school to become a registered nurse, I had many "aha moments." I also had many of these moments while practicing as a LPN as well as the other roles I held while working in the long-term care setting. I will share these moments with you through the content of this book. Each concept will be presented separately but with a similar foundation that includes a description of the concept, objectives, content related to the concept, and the role of the LPN in implementation of the concept into practice. Each chapter will present a different topic with an overarching connection from chapter to chapter. This book is intended as a resource for LPNs in the work setting. The content is intended to support you in your varied roles while impressing upon you and your colleagues the value you bring to the role of nurse.

References

Administration on Aging (2016) Aging statistics. Retrieved from https://aoa.acl.gov/Aging_Statistics/index.aspx

American Health Care Association (2008) Report of findings 2007 AHCA survey nursing staff vacancy and turnover in nursing facilities. Author, Washington, DC

Centers for Disease Control and Prevention (2016) Long-term care providers and services users in the United States: data from the National Study of Long-Term Care Providers, 2013–2014. Centers for Disease Control and Prevention, Atlanta, GA

Deutschman MT (2005) An enthnographic study of nursing home culture to define organizational realities of culture change. J Health Hum Serv Adm 28(2):246–281

Egenes K (2009) History of nursing. Jones and Bartlett Publishers, LLC, Sudbury, MA

Hockenberry J, Becker E (2016) How do hospital nurse staffing strategies affect patient satisfaction? ILR Rev 69(4):890–910

Health Resources and Services Administration (2004) Supply, demand, and use of licensed practical nurses. Retrieved from http://bhpr.hrsa.gov/healthworkforce/reports/supplydemanduselpn.pdf

Kruschke C (2006) The Eden Alternative and Rosebud Nursing Center: does the Eden Alternative improve resident outcomes in a long term care setting? UMI Database, AAT 3240833

Li S, Pittman P, Han X, Lowe T (2017) Nurse-related clinical non-licensed personnel in U.S. hospitals and their relationship with nurse staffing levels. Health Serv Res 52(Supplement 1):422–436

National League for Nursing (2014) A vision for recognition of the role of licensed practical/vocational nurses in advancing the nation's health. National League for Nursing, Washington, DC

Niles N (2014) Basics of the U.S. health care system. Jones and Bartlett Learning, Burlington, MA

Nursingdegreeguide.org (2017) History of nursing in the United States. Retrieved from http://www.nursingdegreeguide.org/articles/general/history_of_nursing_in_the_united_states/

Ragsdale V, McDougall GJ (2008) The changing face of long-term care: looking at the past decade. Issues Ment Health Nurs 29:992–1001

The Health-Care System Related to the Aging Population

2

2.1 Description

This chapter focuses on the health-care system programs and services available to the older adult population. Emerging services are also explored based on current health-care trends including the Affordable Care Act.

2.2 Objectives

1. Identify different health-care systems and the role of each in providing health-care services to the older adult population.
2. Compare and contrast the health-care systems related to health-care service options:
   (a) Acute care
   (b) Long-term care
   (c) Home health care
3. Identify the trends in the environment of the aging population across the continuum of care.
4. Identify variations and complexity of care the LPN will encounter in the future in the various practice settings.

2.3 Health-Care Systems

When we consider health-care systems and what is meant by health-care systems, the first step is to identify what a health-care system is. According to the World Health Organization (2017), a health-care system provides services to a variety of individuals whenever and wherever those services are needed. For our discussion we will define any health-care system related to our aging population as providing

© Springer International Publishing AG 2018
C. Kruschke, *Leadership Skills for Licensed Practical Nurses Working with the Aging Population*, https://doi.org/10.1007/978-3-319-69862-5_2

services wherever and whenever the elder needs those services. This includes the hospital setting, long-term care setting, and home health and hospice as well as palliative care.

2.3.1 Acute Care

The acute care setting provides a variety of services to a variety of individuals at the time they need those services within a geographic area. While this is not a more global definition, within the context of how health care is delivered in the United States, this is a good definition of a health-care system. When we consider the aging population, the services become more focused with services including the emergency department for emergent issues, intensive care unit for emergent issues as well as exacerbation of chronic issues requiring more intense care, medical/surgical care, rehabilitation services, imaging services, lab services, and surgical services. The services provided can be short term or long term depending on the needs of the patient.

The acute care industry includes any medical treatment that is provided on a short-term basis. This is usually as a result of an acute illness, injury, or surgery. Care is usually provided in the hospital setting on a short-term basis.

The acute care setting has undergone dramatic changes as the length of stay has been reduced dramatically to reduce health-care costs. Care levels have also changed as the very ill individuals remain in the acute care setting, while those below the subacute standard are moved to subacute facilities or, if possible, returned home for further care from home health-care agency personnel. The development of new surgical procedures including increased numbers of transplants has also altered the hospital setting as the type of patient admitted changes. The number of hospitals has continued to decline as the length of stay has declined, and the economy has also taken a decline. Hospitals face a myriad of changes including reduction in reimbursement, patients unable to pay for services, and government regulations. This has resulted in hospitals needing to change their business structure to become more efficient with less reimbursement dollars.

There are a variety of hospital services provided including intensive care, emergency care, rehab services, and surgical services. Additional services to the aging population that might be provided include:

1. Mental health services
2. Medical/surgical services
3. Other specialty services such as cardiac, oncology, or orthopedic services

There are a variety of hospital types providing specialized services:
According to the American Hospital Association (2017a), there are 5564 registered hospitals in the United States. This number can be further scrutinized based on the type of hospital including:

- Community hospitals (both for-profit and nonprofit)
- Government hospitals
- Specialty hospitals such as:
  - Orthopedic
  - Cardiac
  - Cancer Treatment
- Teaching hospitals
- Long-term care hospitals providing extended services (American Hospital Association 2017b)
- Critical access hospitals located in rural areas (Department of Health and Human Services 2016)
- Urgent care centers

Community hospitals are those hospitals not considered to be part of the federal government and provide a variety of services to the public including the aging population (American Hospital Association 2017a). **Government hospitals** are owned and operated by the state or federal government. **Specialty hospitals** provide care that is specialized to a specific care area where the hospital excels. These might include orthopedic hospitals, cardiac care hospitals, or hospitals specializing in cancer treatment (Guterman 2006). **Teaching hospitals** provide educational opportunities for medical students. These hospitals are often associated with universities with medical programs requiring clinical placement. **Long-term acute care hospitals** have developed to meet the growing need for acute care services that go beyond the acute phase of an illness or traumatic injury. **Urgent care centers** provide "walk-in" services to consumers in need of medical care who are unable to see their PCP. This service is intended to reduce the number of nonemergency medical care patients walking into hospital emergency rooms to receive care, impacting the ability to meet the needs of all patients who come to the emergency room.

2.3.2   Long-Term Care

2.3.2.1 Nursing Homes

Nursing homes were developed to meet the needs of a growing older adult population no longer able to care for themselves. This need resulted in the development of care homes in order to achieve economies of scale in terms of care providers. With more older adults in one location, the provision of care became more efficient and effective from the perspective of cost.

From these beginnings, long-term care or, specifically, nursing homes evolved into care facilities with an emphasis toward caring for the elderly from admission until death. The need for outpatient rehabilitation services changed the long-term care setting as nursing homes took up the challenge of providing this type of care when acute care settings began looking for alternative settings for patients in need of rehabilitative services. Third-party payers welcomed this shift as cost for care declined when these patients shifted from the acute care setting to the long-term care setting. Nursing homes continue to evolve to meet the needs of their residents including subacute care, rehabilitation, and care of individuals under the age of 65.

Nursing homes may exist as free-standing entities or be attached to a hospital either through bricks and mortar or through an affiliation based on ownership. There are hospital systems in the United States that also own nursing homes. This provides a conduit for the hospital system to care for older adults within their own system.

2.3.2.2 Assisted Living

With the introduction of assisted living homes, patients needing intermediate nursing care were discharged from nursing homes to assisted living if they were able to pay for the services themselves. Assisted living homes provide a variety of services depending on the needs of the patients, who are often called residents. Services include meal preparation, housekeeping services, and laundry services. Additionally, residents are provided assistance with activities as needed. Many assisted living facilities only admit residents who pay with private funds, making these facilities very lucrative in terms of return on investment. There are also assisted living facilities that do admit individuals who have coverage through private insurance or are Medicaid recipients. In these cases, the private insurance company or the local government entity that oversees Medicaid funds will work on an agreement regarding payment for the care provided to the resident with the coverage.

2.3.2.3 RCAC

Residential care apartment complexes provide a variety of services to individuals residing in the complex based on the individual's specific needs. Services can include meal preparation, housekeeping services, laundry services, and/or assistance with activities of daily living. This is considered an assisted living environment where the individuals live in their own apartments.

2.3.2.4 Home Care and Hospice Services

Home health-care agencies have grown from the late 1800s. While the acute care setting has not allowed for medical staff to really know their patients beyond their current medical needs, home health care has provided this well-rounded, holistic care to patients in their own homes. Additionally, home health-care agencies were able to delegate tasks to other care providers in order to achieve better economies of scale. For example, household tasks are delegated to home health aides, while activities of daily living are able to be delegated to home health personal aides trained to provide these types of services. This has provided the home health nurse to focus on the medical needs of the patients while seeing more patients.

2.3.2.5 Independent Living

Independent living environments include private homes, private apartments, and retirement communities.

2.4 Payer Sources for Health-Care Systems

2.4.1 Hospitals

Hospitals contract for payment with private insurance companies for payment. Hospitals tend to contract with multiple private insurance companies in order to increase their overall reimbursement and to increase the percentage of patients who might use their services.

The government is the largest payer source and is considered a third-party payer. However, the government determines the payment the hospital will receive rather than negotiating a price. The new payment system, Prospective Payment System (PPS), has altered the landscape as acute care facilities find ways to become more efficient and effective with tightened payment structures. The current payment system, PPS, requires hospitals to bill for services based on diagnosis-related groups (DRGs), which provide the maximum payment hospitals can receive for specific services provided. While the government is the largest third-party payer for hospital reimbursement, the government is not necessarily the highest paying group. With the implementation of "never events," Medicare no longer pays for, or pays reduced rates, for certain events that occur in a hospital such as infections and falls. More will be discussed regarding payment sources later in this text.

The number of hospitals has continued to decline as the length of stay has declined and the economy has also taken a decline. Hospitals face a myriad of changes including reduction in reimbursement, patients unable to pay for services, and government regulations. This has resulted in hospitals needing to change their business structure to become more efficient with less reimbursement dollars.

2.4.2 Nursing Homes

Nursing homes admit individuals with a variety of payer sources include Medicare, Medicaid, VA benefits, private insurance, and private funds. Private insurance companies work with the nursing homes to contract services at a specific daily rate. Medicare and Medicaid base reimbursement on resource utilization groups (RUGs), which are similar to DRGs in the acute care setting. The government sets the rate for each RUG group.

Long-term care includes a variety of payer sources:

1. Private pay
2. Private insurance
3. Medicare
4. Medicaid
5. Veteran's benefits

Nursing homes contract for payment with private insurance companies for payment. Nursing homes will contract with multiple private insurance companies in order to increase their overall reimbursement and to increase the percentage of patients who might use their services.

The government is the largest payer source and is considered a third-party payer. However, the government determines the payment the nursing home will receive rather than negotiating a price. The new payment system, Perspective Payment System (PPS), has altered the landscape as nursing homes find ways to become more efficient and effective with tightened payment structures. The current payment system, PPS, requires nursing homes to bill for services based on Resource Utilization Groups (RUGs), as discussed previously. More will be discussed regarding payment sources later in this book.

Nursing homes have seen an increase in the number of individuals who do not have a payer source, especially those individuals under the age of 65 and ineligible for government funding. This has resulted in nursing homes no longer being able to sustain themselves. Government funding has also declined as payment structures tighten due to a variety of reasons including the new Prospective Payment System (PPS), the economic decline, and the need for the government to cut spending in order to reduce the overall deficit.

The regulatory climate of the nursing home setting has continued to change the "look" of the nursing home from homes exclusively for the older adult in need of care to homes that encompass adult care from age 18 upward. As adult individuals of all ages need more medically complex care, the nursing home environment changes to meet those needs at the subacute as well as the skilled levels of care.

Finally, with changing regulations and third-party payers scrutinizing care at all levels, nursing homes have also had to rise to these challenges and determine new ways of providing care that embrace a more holistic approach rather than only focusing on the medical model of care. Culture change is rapidly changing the face of health care regardless of the level of care.

2.4.3   Assisted Living

The government payments for Medicare and Medicaid did not truly embrace this change in every state, resulting in many older adults without personal funds being relegated to nursing homes regardless of level of care.

2.4.4   RCACs

Payment sources for RCACs are the same as discussed under assisted living. Payer sources include private funds and Medicaid funding.

2.4.5   Independent Living

Services in private homes and private apartments can be contracted privately with private funds. If an individual requires home health or hospice services, funding can include private funding, private health insurance, and government funding. Home health and hospice services will be discussed separately.

2.4.6   Home Health and Hospice

Home care/hospice services receive payment from a variety of payer sources including:

- Private pay
- Private insurance
- Medicare
- Medicaid
- Veteran's benefits

Home Care and Hospice Services contract with multiple private insurance companies in order to increase their overall reimbursement and to increase the percentage of patients who might use their services.

The government is the largest payer source and is considered a third-party payer. However, the government determines the payment the home care and hospice agencies will receive rather than negotiating a price. The new payment system, prospective payment system, has altered the landscape as home care and hospice agencies find ways to become more efficient and effective with tightened payment structures. The PPS system also defined levels of service as part of the reimbursement process with home health care receiving lower reimbursement levels resulting in a more defined delegation process to meet the regulatory and reimbursement requirements. Home health care has seen a decline in reimbursement rates as the government has strived to reduce costs.

Home health care provides a continuation of care provided at the acute care level or subacute care level by coordinating care in the home setting. Patients being discharged with home health services receive those services without loss of care as the home health agencies fill the gap between inpatient and outpatient services.

Hospice services are provided based on need and are ordered by the primary care physician. Criteria for hospice services vary by state. Variation includes the amount of services provided, where the services will be provided, and the length of time the services will be provided.

2.5   Models of Care to Meet the Needs of the Aging Population

There are a variety of services that have been developed to meet the needs of the aging population. We have already looked at different settings where care might be provided. In addition to the care settings we reviewed, older adults have the opportunity to participate in a variety of programs to meet their needs based on specific criteria for each service.

2.5.1   Programs for All-Inclusive Care for the Elderly (PACE)

This is an optional program under the Medicare and Medicaid programs (Medicaid. gov 2017; Medicare.gov 2017). The program is intended to keep the older adult in their home for as long as possible. Services are provided in the home, at specific PACE organizations as part of day programs, or as an inpatient in another health-care setting. Each PACE center provides services intended to meet the needs of each client. A variety of health-care providers either work for PACE or are contracted through a PACE program to ensure services are provided. Services include the following:

- Adult day care
- Recreational therapy
- Home care
- Hospital care
- Nursing home care
- Therapy services including occupational and physical therapies
- Short-term stay in rehabilitation center or nursing home rehabilitation unit
- Emergency care
- Lab/imaging services
- Meals both at the day care and sent to the home
- Dental care
- Primary care as well as specialty services
- Preventative care
- Nutritional services
- Social services
- Medications
- Transportation to PACE programs and other services

To qualify for PACE services, the following criteria must be met:

- Age 55 and older
- Chronic care needs
- Certified as needing nursing home placement
- Able to live safely in the community
- Resides in an area with PACE services (Medicare.gov, 2017, para 5; National PACE Association, 2017)

If the older adult receives Medicare and Medicaid, the PACE program is available to them free of charge. If the older adult receives Medicare but not Medicaid, the PACE program is available for a monthly fee including payment of a premium under Medicare Part D. In addition, if the individual is not receiving either Medicare or Medicaid, they can join the PACE program for a monthly fee.

Individuals receiving services under the PACE program may be admitted to a hospital or long-term care home and continue to receive PACE services. The PACE program will work with the organization to ensure care is provided based on the facility criteria as well as the PACE program criteria. Each state with a PACE program will have their own program providers. The National PACE Association provides additional information beneficial to potential recipients and providers through their website at http://www.npaonline.org/about-npa. Not every state has a PACE program, while other states have more than one PACE program. You can learn more about your state and if there is a PACE program through the National PACE Association website PACE locator page, http://www.npaonline.org/pace-you/find-pace-program-your-neighborhood.

2.5.2   Nurses Improving Care to Older Adults (NICHE)

Nurses Improving Care to Older Adults (NICHE) is a nurse-run program providing education, evidence-based protocols, and support to organizations wanting to offer care services to older adults (NICHE 2017). The NICHE program has several guiding principles associated with the services provided including:

- Implementation of best practices at the bedside that are evidence-based in the provision of care to the aging population
- Supports best practices in the care of the aging population including:
  - Pain management
  - Reduction and elimination of pressure ulcers
  - Avoidance of adverse medication situations
  - Treatment of delirium
  - Management of urinary incontinence
  - Reduction and elimination of falls
- Supports patient-centered and family-centered environments supportive of the older adult and family members
- A practice environment that promotes autonomy for the older adult as well as the staff who care for the older adult that includes interdisciplinary collaboration and resources specific to the aging population (NICHE 2017)

In addition to the guiding principles, NICHE is also associated with two nursing models of care including the Geriatric Resource Nurse (GRN) model and an Acute Care of the Elderly Medical-Surgical Unit (ACE Unit) (NICHE 2017, para 2 and para 6).

The GRN model of care is intended to promote a better understanding of the care of the aging population beginning with the bedside nurse. The goal is for the bedside nurse to be trained by GRNs to understand and treat specific geriatric syndromes and develop protocols that can be established both on the unit and system-wide. The GRN model has proven effective in developing bedside nurses with an improved perception of caring for the aging population (NICHE 2017).

The Acute Care of the Elderly Medical-Surgical Unit (ACES) is intended to transform a unit or a group of rooms on a unit to include specific interventions that are intended to improve the outcomes of the aging population served on that specific unit. Goals associated with this unit include:

- Environmental adaptations such as nonglare flooring
- Education of staff specific to the aging population
- Development of an interdisciplinary team with a focus on specific geriatric syndromes (NICHE 2017)

2.5.3   Guided Care

Guided care is a model of care meeting the care needs of medically complex older adults with comorbidities. This model of care was developed at John Hopkins University in response to the aging older adult population. This model promotes specialized education of a registered nurse who then works with physicians and other caregivers to provide additional support for those patients considered most in need of these specialized services. This is especially important for primary care practices to develop. Patients are monitored more closely, and provided additional support in the following areas:

- Education of patients and family members
- Promotion of patient autonomy
- Coordination of all health-care providers associated with each patient
- Promotion of smooth transitions between health-care facilities
- Determining community resources that would benefit the aging patient (John Hopkins Bloomberg School of Public Health 2013)

The Guided Care website provides a variety of resources that can be used to help practices implement guided care. These resources can be found at http://guidedcare. org/resources.asp.

2.5.4   Medical Home Model of Care

The Medical Home Model of Care is made up of a variety of providers including doctors, nurses, pharmacists, nutritionists, and other practitioners in the provision of care to patients. This integration of services responds to care complexity. The goal of the medical home model of care is to increase the ability of the practitioners to meet the needs of patients through extended office hours and increased communication including the use of email, website links available to patients, as well as increased use of conference calls to discuss patient issues. Medical homes are as unique as the providers who participate in this model. Each provider has immediate access to patient information that allows for a more comprehensive approach to patient care. In addition, this model promotes cost savings through reduction in duplication of services and promotion of care coordination that is patient-centered (National Conference of State Legislatures 2012; Patient-Centered Primary Care Collaborative 2017).

2.5.5 Transitional Care Models

This program is geared to the older adult with comorbidities including at least five chronic conditions transitioning from one care environment to another. This model is an evidence-based solution to the challenges related to comorbidities and is a nurse-led initiative. This model has the primary goals including the following:

- Development of a collaborative relationship between health-care providers related to the older adult transitioning from one care environment to another care environment or between providers
- Development of a collaborative relationship between the older adult and care providers
- Increasing communication between the older adult and all care providers. Increasing communication between care providers related to the provision of care to the older adult
- Increased follow-up support to the older adult following transition from one care environment to another or between providers
- Development of programs and services to fill care gaps as the older adult transitions from one care environment to another or between providers (Hirschman et al. 2015)
- Reduce rehospitalizations and visits to the emergency room resulting in reduction in patient deaths and health-care costs
- Increase in patient satisfaction (Coalition for Evidence-Based Policy 2015)

2.5.6 Culture Change

Culture change is the movement to improve the care of the aging population through the embracement of person-directed care. According to the Pioneer Network, culture change revolves around the values of "relationship, choice, dignity, respect, self-determination and purposeful living" (Pioneer Network 2017, para 2). You will learn more about this movement in Chapter 10. Developing a Culture Change Person-Centered Environment.

2.6 Services to Meet the Needs of the Aging Population

In addition to the models described, additional services are offered through community, state, and federal initiatives. A sampling of these services is included in Table 2.1.

Table 2.1 Sample aging population services

Administration on Aging
Office on Aging
Commission on Aging
Meals on Wheels
Senior citizen centers
Health screening through community programs
Family caregiver support programs
Alzheimer's Association

2.7   The Role of the LPN in Understanding the Complexity of Care Related to the Aging Population

The LPN has an important role in understanding the complexity of care related to the aging population. Nurses have a responsibility to know what services the older adult will need outside of the care setting they are currently residing in. This includes both registered nurses (RNs) and licensed practical nurses (LPNs). Consider where you are working at this time. Regardless of the care environment, if you have an older adult who is transitioning from one unit to another, from one care environment to another care environment, or from one care environment to home care services, it is the responsibility of the care team completing the transfer to ensure the older adult will have the services necessary to meet their needs. The LPN needs to know what services are currently being offered in their community. You need to investigate the services offered through your own research or ask other members of the care team to share information for your community. We have a responsibility to our aging population to understand their needs and then find the support the older adult will need in order to receive the services they need and want.

For the LPN working in the long-term care setting, this is a critical element to understand. When we transfer a resident to the hospital or another care environment, we need to ensure all the paperwork is correct to make sure the recipient of our resident understands their care needs and can make the best decisions possible with the older adult. For example, when we transfer a resident to the hospital, we need to complete the transfer paperwork including all current orders and what precipitated the transfer. In addition, we should take the time to call the receiving hospital emergency department and speak to a nurse and share the critical information necessary. This dual approach ensures the information we need to share reaches the correct person. I cannot tell you the number of times I transferred a resident to the hospital only to have the paperwork get lost in transit. Taking the time to make a phone call to the receiving hospital ensured the emergency staff had information critical to the care of the resident I sent. Additionally, they knew who to call to receive copies of any paperwork sent but not received.

This approach is also important when transferring a resident to another care environment permanently. For example, when I transferred a resident to an assisted living home, we expected someone from the home to visit the resident in our nursing home so they could meet the resident and learn more about the resident. Then, at the time of the transfer, the paperwork was completed, and I called the receiving home to discuss the resident and their care needs. This way, questions could be asked pertinent to the care of the resident, making the transition smooth. Paperwork was sent via fax and an additional copy sent as a hard copy. We have a responsibility to make sure the receiving home or other provider has the capability of caring for the individual being transferred. While we cannot stop a resident from discharging to a care environment of their preference, we have an obligation to understand where they are going and whether or not the care environment they are going to can meet their needs. If the care environment cannot meet their needs, the care team at your nursing home must provide education to the resident related to the transfer so the resident can make an informed decision along with their representative. As a licensed practical nurse (LPN), I have made these phone calls based on the decisions of the care team regarding transfers and discharges. I have also participated in the education of residents who were at risk of being discharged to an unsafe environment.

References

American Hospital Association (2017a) Fast facts on US hospitals. Retrieved from http://www.aha.org/research/rc/stat-studies/fast-facts.shtml

American Hospital Association (2017b) Long-term care hospitals (LTCHs). Retrieved from http://www.aha.org/advocacy-issues/postacute/ltach/index.shtml

Coalition for Evidence-Based Policy (2015) Transitional care model – top tier. Retrieved from http://evidencebasedprograms.org/1366-2/transitional-care-model-top-tier

Department of Health and Human Services (2016) Critical access hospital. Retrieved from https://www.cms.gov/Outreach-and-Education/Medicare-Learning-Network-MLN/MLNProducts/downloads/CritAccessHospfctsht.pdf

Guterman S (2006) Specialty hospitals: a problem or a symptom? Health Affairs 25(1):95–105

Hirschman K, Shaid E, McCauley K, Pauly M, Naylor M (2015) Continuity of care: the transitional care model. Online J Issues Nurs 20(2):1

John Hopkins Bloomberg School of Public Health (2013) Guided care. Comprehensive primary care for complex patients. Retrieved from http://guidedcare.org/about-us.asp

Medicaid.gov (2017) Program of all-inclusive care for the elderly. Retrieved from https://www.medicaid.gov/medicaid/ltss/pace/index.html

Medicare.gov (2017). PACE. Retrieved from https://www.medicare.gov/your-medicare-costs/help-paying-costs/pace/pace.html

National Conference of State Legislatures (2012) The medical home model of care. Retrieved from http://www.ncsl.org/research/health/the-medical-home-model-of-care.aspx

National PACE Association (2017). Understanding PACE. Retrieved from http://www.npaonline.org/sites/default/files/PDFs/3%20PACE%20Fact%20Sheet%20DRAFT%201.pdf

NICHE (2017) Program overview. Retrieved from http://www.nicheprogram.org/program-overview/

Patient-Centered Primary Care Collaborative (2017) Defining the medical home. Retrieved from https://www.pcpcc.org/about/medical-home

Pioneer Network (2017). Defining culture change. Retrieved from https://www.pioneernetwork.net/culturechange/what-is-culture-change/

World Health Organization (2017) Health systems. Retrieved from http://www.who.int/topics/health_systems/en/

Regulatory Compliance and the Role of the Licensed Practical Nurse

3

3.1 Description

This chapter focuses on regulatory requirements for all Licensed Practical Nurses (LPNs) based on the nurse practice act for each state. This chapter also looks at the regulatory requirements for health-care providers including hospitals, nursing homes, assisted living homes, and home health agencies. LPNs need to understand their own scope of practice as well as the requirements of licensing for the health-care entity they work for in order to ensure all rules and regulations are followed.

3.2 Objectives

1. Review the rules and regulations pertaining to the licensed practical nurse including scope of practice.
2. Review regulatory compliance and the role of the LPN.
3. Nursing practice standards for the licensed practical nurse.
4. Standards of Practice and Educational Competencies of Graduates of Practical/Vocational Nursing Programs.
5. Regulatory compliance for health-care entities including hospitals, nursing homes, assisted living homes, and home health agencies.

3.3 Review the Rules and Regulations Pertaining to the Licensed Practical Nurse Including Scope of Practice

This is a good point to review the nurse practice act from each state. Chapter 12 provides a listing for each state where you can obtain information for your own state or another state of interest. This chapter also provides a brief synopsis of the nurse

© Springer International Publishing AG 2018   23
C. Kruschke, *Leadership Skills for Licensed Practical Nurses Working with the Aging Population*, https://doi.org/10.1007/978-3-319-69862-5_3

practice act. I would like to thank Deborah Leon for researching the nurse practice act in each state and providing the information for this book. Table 3.1 provides a listing of the boards of nursing for each state and specific territories of the United States.

In addition to learning more about your nurse practice act, we will explore the overarching scope of practice for most LPNs/LVNs in the United States. This information is not intended to be inclusive but provides a basic overview impacting the practicing LPN/LVN. As I stated in the introduction, I was a LPN for many years. The LPN is trained as a licensed nurse with specific limitations that are associated with the training received as well as taking into consideration the training not received in an accredited program. The LPN/LVN is considered to be an extension of the registered nurse with specific limitations in practice including assessment and nursing diagnosis. The LPN/LVN is able to collect information that can be reported to the physician, registered nurse, advanced practice nurse, or physician's assistant. However, the data collected cannot be used by the LPN/LVN to provide an actual assessment. This is based on the limitations of the scope of practice. In addition, while the registered nurse is able to provide a nursing diagnosis through the assessment process, the LPN/LVN is not able to do the same. Again, the LPN/LVN is limited to the collection of information.

The National Federation for Licensed Practical Nurses adopted standards of practice for the LPN in 1961 (National Federation of Licensed Practical Nurses, Inc. 2003). The LPN/LVN is a critical member of the health-care team. Depending on the work environment, the LPN/LVN will take on a variety of roles, which we will discuss later in this chapter. As part of these varied roles, the LPN/LVN is trained to collect information as part of the planning process and report the data collected to the appropriate member of the team. Then, this data is used to implement the plan developed for each patient. Then, the implemented plan is evaluated to determine if the plan is working. If the plan is not working, the LPN/LVN will collect additional data, develop a new plan, and evaluate the plan at some point in the future (National Federation of Licensed Practical Nurses, Inc. 2003).

The National Council of State Boards of Nursing (NCSBN) has periodically convened focus groups to review the LPN/LVN scope of practice based on actual practice tasks performed and knowledge base. From this information, the NCSBN has determined there are states where the LPN/LVN works outside their scope of practice while in other states the LPN/LVN works below their scope of practice. The common practice standards for most states include data collection as part of the planning process, implementation of the plan, and evaluation of the plan. From these common tasks, the LPN/LVN will have additional tasks associated with their license depending on the state they are practicing in. In some states the nurse practice act does not allow for LPNs/LVNs to perform higher functions such as blood transfusions or dialysis, while other states do allow for these tasks to be performed if there is a RN monitoring the LPN/LVN. However, the level of monitoring varies significantly across the country. As a LPN, I was required to report to the RN in charge. However, I had many experiences of working on a shift with other LPNs, and the RN in charge was only available by phone. This posed a huge issue for us nurses working on units without the ability to have the RN join us on the unit to

Table 3.1 State Boards of Nursing

State	Website
Alabama	https://www.abn.alabama.gov/
Alaska	https://www.commerce.alaska.gov/web/cbpl/ ProfessionalLicensing/BoardofNursing.aspx
American Samoa	https://www.ncsbn.org/American%20Samoa.htm
Arizona	http://www.azbn.gov/
Arkansas	http://www.arsbn.org/
California	rn.ca.gov/
Colorado	colorado.gov/pacific/dora/Nursing
Connecticut	ct.gov/dph/cwp/view
Delaware	dpr.delaware.gov/boards/nursing/
District of Columbia	doh.dc.gov/node/
Florida	floridasnursing.gov/
Georgia	sos.ga.gov/index.php/licensing/plb/45
Guam	dphss.guam.gov/content/guam-board-nurse-examiners
Hawaii	cca.hawaii.gov/pvl/boards/nursing/
Idaho	ibn.idaho.gov/
Illinois	www.idfpr.com/profs/Nursing.asp
Indiana	in.gov/pla/nursing.htm
Iowa	nursing.iowa.gov
Kansas	ksbn.org/
Kentucky	kbn.ky.gov
Louisiana	lsbn.state.la.us
Maine	maine.gov/boardofnursing/
Maryland	mbon.maryland.gov/Pages/default.aspx
Massachusetts	mass.gov/eohhs/gov/departments/dph/programs/hcq/dhpl/ nursing/
Michigan	michigan.gov/
Minnesota	nursingboard.state.mn.us/
Mississippi	msbn.ms.gov/Pages/Home.aspx
Missouri	pr.mo.gov/nursing.asp
Montana	nurse.mt.gov
Nebraska	dhhs.ne.gov/publichealth/Pages/crl_nursing_nursingindex.aspx
Nevada	nevadanursingboard.org/
New Hampshire	nh.gov/nursing/
New Jersey	njconsumeraffairs.gov/nur/Pages/default.aspx
New Mexico	nmbon.sks.com/
New York	op.nysed.gov/prof/nurse/
North Carolina	ncbon.com/
North Dakota	ndbon.org/
Northern Mariana Islands	nmicbne.com/
Ohio	nursing.ohio.gov
Oklahoma	ok.gov/nursing/
Oregon	osbn.state.or.us/
Pennsylvania	dos.pa.gov/ProfessionalLicensing/BoardsCommissions/Nursing/ Pages/default.aspx#.VTEYxCFVhBd
Rhode Island	health.ri.gov/for/nurses/index.php
South Carolina	llr.state.sc.us/pol/nursing
South Dakota	doh.sd.gov/boards/nursing/
Tennessee	tn.gov/health/topic/nursing-board
Texas	bon.texas.gov

(continued)

Table 3.1 (continued)

State	Website
Utah	dopl.utah.gov/licensing/nursing.html
Vermont	sec.state.vt.us
Virgin Islands	thevibnl.org
Virginia	dhp.virginia.gov/nursing/
Washington	doh.wa.gov/LicensesPermitsandCertificates/NursingCommission. aspx
West Virginia	wvrnboard.wv.gov/Pages/default.aspx
Wisconsin	dsps.wi.gov/Default.aspx
Wyoming	nursing-online.state.wy.us/

respond to questions or concerns. This was an acceptable practice for many years and, in some cases, is still an acceptable practice that can lead to issues for the LPN.

3.4   The Role of the LPN

While your role as a licensed practical nurse is limited in terms of scope of practice, you are still an integral member of the leadership team. As such, you have a responsibility to adhere to the regulations associated with the care environment you work with. Take the following steps to ensure you understand your role:

1. Review the nurse practice act for the LPN in your state.
2. Review the state and federal guidelines for your health-care facility.

As a licensed practical nurse (LPN) or licensed vocational nurse (LVN), you are a member of your leadership team. While your scope of practice differentiates you from the registered nurse (RN) and the certified nursing assistant (CNA), you are responsible for directing the care of the patients you provide care to under the supervision of a RN. In the acute care setting, the RN may delegate tasks to you such as medication administration, wound care, and oversight of the CNAs. In the long-term care setting, you may be delegated the task of overseeing an entire unit including the care of the residents and oversight of the certified nursing assistants (CNAs) including delegation of care tasks to the CNAs. As a former LPN, I understand the restrictions of licensing for the LPN/LVN. However, I also understand the rationale for these restrictions. Our education is not as extensive as the RN but provides us with the information we need to work in conjunction with a RN.

3.5   Nursing Practice Standards for the Licensed
Practical Nurse

Each state has its own rules and regulations related to the licensing and scope of practice for the LPN/LVN. These requirements translate into the educational competencies expected of all graduates of practical/vocational nursing programs. The National Association for Licensed Practical Nurses (2007) has developed Standards of Practice and Educational Competencies of Graduates of Practical/Vocational Nursing Programs. The LPN is required to exhibit professional behavior in all aspects of the nursing process. This includes the adherence to ethical and legal practices. The LPN is expected to maintain the knowledge and competencies to remain current in all practices outlined in their specific state scope of practice. The LPN must exhibit appropriate communication skills across the health-care continuum as well as communicating to patients and family members. This includes both written and oral communication. The LPN is also expected to collect relevant data for analysis in order to provide the highest level of care possible based on the analysis of the data collected. The data collected is documented in the patient's permanent record and reported to the appropriate practitioner and team members to establish the appropriate plan of care. This plan of care is developed in conjunction with the registered nurse (RN) and in collaboration with the interdisciplinary team as necessary in the provision of quality care. The LPN is expected to provide care through an empathetic approach maintaining the patient's autonomy and allowing for the highest level of comfort and functionality. Additionally, the LPN is charged with the responsibility to provide a safe environment for the patient both physically and psychosocially. The LPN is also charged with the responsibility of delegation of care to certified nursing assistants or personal care assistants with the scope of practice of that role. The LPN who delegates tasks to certified nursing assistants or personal care assistants is responsible for ensuring those tasks are completed appropriately. The LPN is required to be fiscally responsible through cost-effective approaches to the provision of care (National Association for Practical Nurse Education and Service, Inc. 2007).

The National Council of State Boards of Nursing, Inc. (2005) developed a white paper addressing the scope of practice of LPNs/LVNs. According to the research completed for this paper, the state boards of nursing were queried regarding the role of the LPN/LVN in each state. Through this process the following results were reported:

- Most states reported that LPNs/LVNs should not independently develop plans of care except under the guidance of a registered nurse (RN). A change in the plan of care also must be approved by the RN unless the LPN/LVN received additional training related to the care planning process.
- The majority of boards of nursing indicated the LPN/LVN would not be able to complete phone triage with patients and that all abnormal findings must be reported to the patient's physician or the RN.
- Many of the boards of nursing reported the LPN/LVN could provide teaching to patients; however, their scope of practice did not allow for the LPN/LVN to develop the teaching independently. The development of the education needs to take place under the supervision of the RN or the RN must develop the education. The RN can then delegate the teaching aspect to the LPN/LVN.
- Many of the states reported that LPNs/LVNs were able to look at lab values and other data to determine if the data is within the normal limits. The plan of care is updated or changed under the supervision of the RN or physician depending on the lab results. LPNs/LVNs have the capacity to add to the care plan.
- In terms of comparing a patient's psychological status or potential for violence to the norm, many of the state boards of nursing reported LPNs/LVNs needed

additional education to complete this task and needed to work under the supervision of the RN or physician in these cases.

- The majority of boards of nursing determined the LPN/LVN would need additional training to administer blood products. However, the LPN/LVN would be able to monitor blood transfusions in the majority of states.
- State boards of nursing varied a great deal related to IV therapy and the role of the LPN/LVN. Most states reported the LPN/LVN could assess the IV site and flow rate of the IV as well as give medications through a peripheral line. Beyond that, states were varied in terms of the role of the LPN in IV therapy.
- In most states LPNs/LVNs were not able to develop an independent practice; the role of the LPN/LVN was able to expand.
- LPNs/LVNs are not allowed to make decisions independent of the RN or physician in most states. However, through delegation, LPNs/LVNs are able to make decisions based on their ability and the delegation process.
- The majority of states reported that LPNs/LVNs are not able to complete an assessment but are able to collect data related to the patient and share the information with the RN or physician. Decision-making based on the data collected is based on the LPNs/LVNs scope of practice within each state.
- The LPN/LVN is able to delegate tasks as appropriate in a majority of the states. However, the LPN/LVN is required to ensure the individual who is being delegated to must have the knowledge, skills, and abilities to complete the task delegated to them (National Council of State Boards of Nursing, Inc. 2005).

The overarching results of this paper indicated each LPN/LVN needs to review their state's nurse practice act to determine their specific scope of practice.

3.6   Regulatory Compliance for Health-Care Entities Including Hospitals, Nursing Homes, Assisted Living Homes, and Home Health Agencies

The federal government oversees the regulatory requirements for all health-care entities including hospitals, nursing homes, assisted living homes, home health agencies, hospice, and palliative care. Reviewing the requirements is beneficial.

Each state has its own regulatory requirements for health-care providers. While we cannot include the information associated with each state, please review the listing of regulatory agencies for each state included in the Table 3.2.

3.6.1   Hospitals

The State Operations Manual, Appendix A: Survey Protocol, Regulations and Interpretive Guidelines for Hospitals can be retrieved from https://www.cms.gov/Regulations-and-Guidance/Guidance/Manuals/downloads/som107ap_a_hospitals.pdf

Hospitals are certified for Medicare/Medicaid through the Centers for Medicare and Medicaid Services (CMS). This certification is necessary to receive payment from the government.

Table 3.2 State regulatory agencies

State	Regulatory agency	URL
Alabama	ADPH Department Of Public Health	www.alabamapublichealth.gov
Alaska	Department of Commerce, Community and Economic Development	www.commerce.alaska.gov
Arizona	AZBN – Arizona Board of Nursing	www.azbn.gov
Arkansas	Arkansas Department of Health	www.healthy.arkansas.gov
California	Department of Consumer Affairs/Online Services	www.dca.ca.gov
Colorado	Department Of Regulatory Agency/Divisions/Profession and Occupations	www.colorado.gov/dora
Connecticut	Department of Public Health	www.ct.gov/dph
Delaware	Division of Professional Regulation	www.dpr.delaware.gov
Florida	Florida Health	www.floridahealth.gov
Georgia	Georgia Department of Community Health GDCH	https://dch.georgia.gov
Hawaii	Department of Commerce and Consumer Affairs/Professional and Vocational Licensing	https://cca.hawaii.gov
Idaho	Department of Health and Welfare/Medical	https//healthandwelfare.idaho.gov
Illinois	Illinois Department of Health	www.dph.illinois.gov
Indiana	Department of Health/Health Care Quality and Regulatory	www.in.gov/isdh
Iowa	State of Iowa – Select Menu – Select Services	www.iowa.gov
Kansas	Department of Health and Environment/Licensing	www.kdheks.gov/health
Kentucky	Cabinet for Health and Family Services	www.chfs.ky.gov
Louisiana	Department of Health/Documents	https//ldh.louisiana.gov
Maine	Department of Health and Human Services	www.maine.gov/dhhs
Maryland	Department of Health	https//health.maryland.gov
Massachusetts	Office of Health and Human Services/Licensing	www.mass.gov/eohhs
Michigan	Department of Licensing and Regulatory Affairs	www.michigan.gov/lara
Minnesota	Department of Health	www.health.state.mn.us
Mississippi	Department of Health	www.msdh.ms.gov
Missouri	Department of Health and Senior Services	www.health.mo.gov
Montana	Department of Public Health and Human Services/Medical	www.dphhs.mt.gov
Nebraska	Department of Health and Human Services/Licensure Unit	www.dhhs.ne.gov
Nevada	Division of Public and Behavioral Health	www.dpbh.nv.gov

(continued)

Table 3.2 (continued)

State	Regulatory agency	URL
New Hampshire	Department of Health and Human Services/Office of Operations Support	www.dhhs.nh.gov
New Jersey	Department of Health	www.nj.gov/health
New Mexico	Regulation and Licensing Department	www.rld.state.mn.us/boards
New York	Department of Health	www.health.ny.gov
North Carolina	Department of Health and Human Services	www.ncdhhs.gov
North Dakota	Department of Health/Health Facilities	www.ndhealth.gov
Ohio	Department of Health/State Agencies/Health	www.odh.ohio.gov
Oklahoma	Department of Health	www.ok.gov/health
Oregon	Department of Human Services	www.oregon.gov/dhs
Pennsylvania	Department of Health	www.health.pa.gov
Rhode Island	Department of Health	www.health.ri.gov
South Carolina	Department of Health and Environment Control	www.scdhec.gov
South Dakota	Department of Health	www.doh.sd.gov
Tennessee	Department of Health	https:tn.gov/health
Texas	Health and Human Services/Doing Business with HHS	www.hhs.texas.gov
Utah	Department of Health	www.health.utah.gov
Vermont	Division of Licensing and Protection/Survey and Certification/Information Facilities and Providers	www.dlp.vermont.gov
Virginia	Department of Health	www.vdh.virginia.gov
Washington	Department of Health	www.doh.wa.gov
West Virginia	Department of Health and Human Resources/Office of Health Facility Licensure and Certification	https//ohflac.wvdhhr.org
Wisconsin	Department of Health Services	www.dhs.wisconsin.gov
Wyoming	Department of Health/Divisions	https//health.wyo.gov

Hospitals may also be Joint Commission (JCAHO) certified. The Joint Commission is a voluntary accreditation program that certifies a variety of providers including hospitals, home care agencies, laboratory services, and nursing homes. According to the JCAHO website, this accreditation is recognized nationwide, and JCAHO is considered "a symbol of quality" (The Joint Commission 2017a, para 1).

3.6.2 Nursing Homes

The State Operations Manual, Appendix PP: Guidance to Surveyors for Long Term Care Facilities can be retrieved from https://www.cms.gov/Regulations-and-Guidance/Guidance/Manuals/downloads/som107ap_pp_guidelines_ltcf.pdf

Nursing homes are certified for Medicare/Medicaid through the Centers for Medicare and Medicaid Services (CMS). This certification is necessary to receive payment from the government.

Nursing homes may also be certified by The Joint Commission. As stated previously, The Joint Commission is a voluntary accreditation program that certifies a variety of providers. According to The Joint Commission website, JCAHO-accredited nursing homes perform better related to specific quality measures as compared to non-accredited nursing homes (The Joint Commission 2017b).

3.6.3   Home Health Agencies

The State Operations Manual, Appendix B: Guidance to Surveyors: Home Health Agencies can be retrieved from https://www.cms.gov/Regulations-and-Guidance/Guidance/Manuals/downloads/som107ap_b_hha.pdf

Home health agencies are certified for Medicare/Medicaid through the Centers for Medicare and Medicaid Services (CMS). This certification is necessary to receive payment from the government.

Home health agencies may also be certified by The Joint Commission. This is a voluntary program home health agencies can participate in. According to The Joint Commission, home health agencies accredited through JACHO have improved outcomes over home health agencies that are not JCAHO accredited including lower rate of emergency room visits and lower readmission rates (The Joint Commission 2017c).

3.6.4   Assisted Living Homes

Assisted living homes are regulated separately by each state rather than national regulations. Understanding the responsibilities of each state is important for all members of leadership including licensed practical nurses. AssistedLiving.com provides the link to each state's licensing and regulatory requirements for assisted living homes. These links can be found at http://www.assistedliving.com/laws-by-state/. Table 3.2 provides a listing of regulatory agencies for each state.

Review the licensing information for your workplace to determine the rules and regulations your facility falls under.

3.7   The Role of the LPN to Maintain Regulatory Compliance

The LPN/LVN works under the supervision of the registered nurse (RN) or physician. The LPN/LVN has a requirement to understand the rules and regulations for themselves as well as the home they work in. Maintaining regulatory compliance is critical in order to continue the operation of the entity they work for. The LPN/LVN works under the supervision of the registered nurse and/or physician regardless of the location. However, this does not mean the LPN/LVN is not responsible for regulatory compliance.

I was a LPN/LVN for many years, and it was my responsibility to ensure the unit I worked on was in compliance with regulations both at the state level and at the federal level. I worked specifically in the nursing home setting and developed my philosophy of regulatory compliance over the course of my experience. Each year the nursing home I worked for was required to have a survey completed to determine if the nursing home was in compliance with the federal guidelines based on the survey manual called the State Operations Manual. Over time I became very familiar with the State Operations Manual as we reviewed the content throughout the year to ensure we were in compliance. I had more experience working with the manual as a nursing home administrator and a director of nursing. However, the belief that all staff should have some knowledge of the rules and regulations related to their role in the nursing home was important. I developed the belief "if you cannot do it when state is in the building, you cannot do it at all" and "if you should be doing it when state is in the building, then you should do it all the time." It was bewildering to me that we would become lax during the course of the year until we were within our window for a state survey, which came between 9 and 18 months after the most recent annual survey. We would become lax and then set about to educate the staff and the rules and regulations and making sure we were doing what we were supposed to be doing. This seemed like a waste of valuable time. My goal became to follow the rules and regulations all year long. I read the State Operations Manual whenever I had a question regarding the rules and regulations. I needed to make sure that staff also understood the rules and regulations and the way to ensure that was happening was to understand them myself and make sure all staff understood them as well.

As a staff nurse, both as a LPN and eventually a RN, it was my responsibility to make sure the unit I was in charge of for a shift was in compliance. This was a requirement for all the nurses working in the organization. Examples of my role as a LPN/LVN ensuring compliance that you need to consider as well include the following. This is not an all-inclusive list. I am sure you can think of many other examples of what needs to be done to remain in compliance:

- When passing medications, I needed to follow the five rights of medication administration including the right medication, the right dose, the right patient, the right time, and the right route. I also needed to use the medication administration record (MAR) with each medication pass despite knowing all of the residents I cared for and the medications they received. I could have passed the medications without using the MAR, but I knew this was not correct.
- When a resident needs to be assessed, I would report the need to the registered nurse (RN), and the RN would complete the assessment. As a LPN, my scope of practice did not allow for me to complete any assessments. Instead, I was able to collect data regarding the resident's status and report my findings to the RN and/ or physician. I then documented the data collection process and the steps I took to report the findings including who I contacted and what I reported. This occurs with falls, wounds, changes of condition, illness, injury, or any other event that is new, is unique, or changes the status of the resident.

- Knocking on the resident's room door is important before entering. Regardless of whether or not state was in the building completing a survey, I made sure to knock on all resident's doors before entering their room. I also made sure the staff working with me on the unit knocked as well. They also did the same for me, reminding me when I forgot to knock on resident doors.
- Each time I received a new order from the physician or nurse practitioner, I contacted the resident's representative to report the change in medication. This was important to do regardless of what the order was for. One of the areas of concern for surveyors is the lack of communication with residents and their representatives. This applies to change of condition or any other issue that arises with the resident.
- Laundry carts used to transport linen and resident clothing should be covered.
- When a resident is on isolation, the staff need to have the appropriate personal protective equipment (PPE) available to wear.
- We need to make sure residents have a choice in an atmosphere of culture change that places the resident at the center of care provided. We need to make sure residents are autonomous throughout the year not just when we are being surveyed. Additional information regarding culture change will come later in this book.
- LPNs/LVNs are expected to advance their knowledge, skills, and abilities in order to maintain their professional level of standing. This includes attending all education provided by the organization you work for and to seek out education outside the organization.

Your role as a LPN/LVN in regulatory compliance is not limited by your standard of practice. On the contrary, regardless of your position in a health-care entity, compliance is your responsibility. We need to work collaboratively to ensure rules and regulations are followed. This is your responsibility. This responsibility belongs to all of us.

References

National Association for Practical Nurse Education and Service, Inc. (2007) Standards of practice and educational competencies of graduates of Practical/Vocational Nursing Programs. National Association for Practical Nurse Education and Service, Inc., Springfield, OH

National Council of State Boards of Nursing, Inc. (2005) Practical nurse scope of practice white paper. National Council of State Boards of Nursing, Inc., Chicago, IL

National Federation of Licensed Practical Nurses, Inc. (2003) Nursing practice standards for the licensed practical/vocational nurse. National Federation of Licensed Practical Nurses, Inc., Raleigh, NC

The Joint Commission (2017a) About the Joint Commission. Retrieved from https://www.joint-commission.org/about_us/about_the_joint_commission_main.aspx

The Joint Commission (2017b) Accreditation for Florida nursing homes. Retrieved from https://www.jointcommission.org/certification/ncc_florida.aspx

The Joint Commission (2017c) Joint Commission accreditation for home health. Retrieved from https://www.jointcommission.org/joint_commission_accreditation_for_home_health/

Fiscal Management and the Role of the LPN (Working in Long-Term Care)

4

4.1 Description

The LPN is required to be fiscally responsible through cost-effective approaches to the provision of care. While the LPN is not required to know finance or financial aspects of health care, knowledge regarding how payment is received and the role of the LPN in ensuring the appropriate payment is able to be billed and received is important. This chapter will provide an overview of how payment is billed and received and the role of the LPN related to fiscal responsibility especially related to documentation.

4.2 Objectives

1. Identify payer systems across the health-care continuum.
2. Review incentive programs provided across the health-care continuum.
3. Fiscal responsibility related to appropriate billing and payment for services provided.
4. Identify the role of the LPN in fiscal management.
5. Review the role of the LPN related to appropriate documentation of patient care.

4.3 Payer System Changes

Nurses need to understand the basics of the payer systems associated with the organization they work at. This does not require an in-depth understanding of finance but a clear understanding of which payment sources are part of the organization and the role of the nurse in fiscal management. This information is part of the regulatory requirements all providers of health care must meet in order to receive payment.

© Springer International Publishing AG 2018
C. Kruschke, *Leadership Skills for Licensed Practical Nurses Working with the Aging Population*, https://doi.org/10.1007/978-3-319-69862-5_4

4.4   Balanced Budget Act of 1997

Reductions in payments to the following providers has been realized since passage of the Balanced Budget Act of 1997. The goal of this budget act was to balance the budget by the year 2002 and included provisions for health care providers as follows:

- Hospitals through development of the prospective payment system. You can learn more about the provisions of this act through the American Hospital Association at http://www.aha.org/advocacy-issues/toolsresources/advisory/96-06/970805-legislative-adv.shtml
- Home Health through the development of the home health prospective payment system. You can learn more about this topic through the Centers for Medicare and Medicaid Services (CMS) at https://www.cms.gov/Medicare/Medicare-Fee-for-Service-Payment/HomeHealthPPS/index.html
- Skilled Nursing Facilities through the development of the prospective payment system. You can learn more about this topic through the Centers for Medicare and Medicaid Services (CMS) at https://www.cms.gov/Medicare/Medicare-Fee-for-Service-Payment/SNFPPS/index.html?redirect=/snfpps

4.5   Centers for Medicare and Medicaid Services (CMS)

The Centers for Medicare and Medicaid Services oversees the Medicare and Medicaid programs as well as other programs to meet the needs of over 100 million people. For health-care providers, understanding Medicare and Medicaid is very important. The Centers for Medicare and Medicaid Services also provides monitoring of health-care agencies to ensure compliance with rules and regulations applicable to that health-care organization. Review the website to learn more about this organization and the benefits of this agency.

4.6   Government Controls

The government is the largest payer source for health care, providing 20% of health-care funding for Medicare and 17% of health-care spending for Medicaid (Centers for Medicare and Medicaid Services 2015).

4.6.1   Medicare

Medicare was first developed in the 1960s during President Johnson's administration and was signed into law at the same time as Medicaid. Medicare was intended to ensure medical coverage for older adults over the age of 65. Initially, Medicare coverage included Medicare A and Medicare B. Medicare A paid for hospitalization and the subsequent care required. Medicare B was related to ancillary costs of medical care not attached to hospitalization such as home health care and medical equipment provided in the home. Additional services covered by Medicare require a qualifying hospital stay. A qualifying hospital stay requires a Medicare recipient to be hospitalized for a 3-day minimum stay. This means the individual must be in a hospital bed for three midnights in a row. Once this occurs, Medicare A benefits will pay for the hospital stay as well as certain services needed beyond the hospital stay if required by a physician and the patient meets all qualifications for the services. These services might include long-term care in a nursing home setting or home health care in a home setting (Medicare.gov, 2017).

4.6.1.1 Coverage

- Medicare, Part A: hospital stays, nursing home stays with a qualifying hospital stay, home health care, hospice care
- Medicare, Part B: physician services, other provider services, home health, durable medical equipment, outpatient care, prevention services (not all services)
- Medicare, Part C: Medicare Advantage Plan for prescription coverage
- Medicare, Part D: Medicare prescription drug plan adds coverage to Medicare Part A and Part B (Medicare.gov, 2017)

The Centers for Medicare and Medicaid Services oversees the Medicare program. You can obtain additional information regarding this program at https://www.medicare.gov/.

4.6.2 Medicaid

Medicaid was first developed in the 1960s during President Johnson's administration and was signed into law at the same time as Medicare. Medicaid was set up to provide health-care services for low-income families including older adults over the age of 65. Coverage for families with children was considered Aid to Families with Dependent Children or AFDC. Individuals under age 65 may now qualify depending on their circumstances. Medicaid pays for services provided based on a predetermined rate for each provider type. Many older adults rely on Medicaid to cover the health-care needs especially if they need services outside the home such as nursing home care (Medicaid.gov, 2017).

The challenge today is to maintain costs while providing the necessary health-care services to each patient. This becomes more difficult as reimbursement rates remain stagnant or decline as costs continue to climb. This has resulted in many health-care providers, such as physicians, refusing to take on any additional patients with Medicare or Medicaid as a payer source. This results in consumers having fewer choices in terms of health-care providers. In some areas of the country, consumers are left with no care providers, especially primary care physicians (Medicaid.gov, 2017).

The Medicaid program is funded by federal dollars as well as state funding. Each state develops a program based on federal guidelines and can amend the program to meet current federal guidelines as well as state guidelines. The Centers for Medicare and Medicaid Services oversee the Medicaid program. If a state wishes to amend its program, the state must apply to the Centers for Medicare and Medicaid Services for approval. Each state determines eligibility, the benefits that will be covered, and the amount providers will be paid (Medicaid.gov, 2017).

The passage of the Affordable Care Act in 2010 has expanded Medicaid coverage and each state is determining level of involvement in the Affordable Care Act. You can review additional information regarding this provision at https://www.medicaid.gov/. The Centers for Medicare and Medicaid Services oversees the Medicaid program. With the current changes being made in Washington D.C. the future of the Affordable Care Act is not guaranteed. Additional government benefits include Veteran's Benefits and Indian Benefits.

4.6.2.1 Veteran's Benefits

The Veterans Benefits Administration was established in 1930. Information is found at US Department of Veterans Affairs, http://www.va.gov/. There are 21.5 million veterans and over 1700 hospitals, clinics, nursing homes, and domiciliaries offering services to veterans. In addition, veterans also use the services of hospitals, clinics, and nursing homes that are not associated with the Veterans Benefits Administration. This means you might have the opportunity to care for veterans in your own healthcare organization (U.S. Department of Veterans Affairs, 2017).

4.6.2.2 Bureau of Indian Affairs

The Bureau of Indian Affairs was established in 1824 to provide services to Native Americans, Indian tribes, and Alaska natives. Services are provided to all federally recognized tribes, which totals 567 representing 1.9 million individuals (U.S. Department of the Interior, 2017). The Bureau of Indian Affairs provides education, health-care services, natural resource management, and economic support services (U.S. Department of Health and Human Services, 2017). Visit the US Department of Health and Human Services website for the Indian Health Services, http://www.ihs.gov/, for additional information or the US Department of the Interior, Indian Affairs, at https://www.bia.gov/index.htm

4.7   Additional Government Controls

The government is the largest payer source for health care and spends a great deal of time developing payment systems and protocols to save money. Understanding some of these payment systems and protocols is beneficial to nurses, including LPNs, especially related to how documentation impacts reimbursement. We will first review some of the payment systems and protocols, and then we will discuss the role of the nurse in understanding these systems and how nurses can impact reimbursement.

4.7.1   Prospective Payment System

The prospective payment system (PPS) was developed based on diagnostic-related groups (DRGs) and resource utilization group (RUGs). These structures put a cap on the amount of money a provider is reimbursed for specific diagnoses. Another structure in place is called the relative value units (RVUs) used by physicians to obtain reimbursement.

4.7.1.1 Diagnostic-Related Groups (DRGs)

Diagnostic-related groups (DRGs) are used in the acute care setting and home health to determine the reimbursement rate for providers. The provider is given a fixed amount of dollars for each DRG. If the provider is able to reduce cost and save money, the provider reaps the benefit of this savings as the payment remains the same. Conversely, if the provider spends more than what is reimbursed, the provider must absorb those costs.

4.7.1.2 Resource Utilization Groups (RUGs)

Resource utilization groups (RUGs) are used in the long-term care setting to determine the reimbursement rate for providers. The provider is given a fixed amount of dollars for each RUG. If the provider is able to reduce cost and save money, the provider reaps the benefit of this savings as the payment remains the same. Conversely, if the provider spends more than what is reimbursed, the provider must absorb those costs. The Centers for Medicare and Medicaid Services has developed reimbursement protocols to save money and make providers of health care more responsible for fiscal management while providing quality care.

4.7.1.3 Relative Value Units (RVUs)

Relative Value Units refer to the services provided by physicians. Each service fee depends on the relative value unit assigned to that service. The fee is based on the resources used to provide the service identified including the physician's care, other support services, and the cost of doing business.

4.7.2   Never Events

Never events were named for situations occurring in the hospital setting determined to be avoidable. These events were able to be identified through historical information provided by hospitals and were also determined to cause harm to patients. The Centers for Medicare and Medicaid Services determined these events were avoidable resulting in loss of reimbursement for the care of the patient that can be attributed to a never event (Centers for Medicare and Medicaid Services, 2008). Additional information regarding never events can be obtained from www. cms.gov. The potential exists for never events to become part of the reimbursement system for the long-term care setting, which will impact reimbursement. Given this potential, understanding never events is important. Table 4.1 provides a list of never events.

Additional information regarding never events can be found at the following websites:

- Agency for Healthcare Research and Quality, http://psnet.ahrq.gov/primer. aspx?primerID=3
- Centers for Medicare and Medicaid Services, https://www.cms.gov/Newsroom/ MediaReleaseDatabase/Press-Releases/2008-Press-Releases-Items/2008-07-313. html

Table 4.1   Never events

Hospital-acquired infections
Development of a stage 3 or stage 4 pressure ulcer after admission to the health-care facility
Surgery or other invasive procedure to the wrong site
Surgery or other invasive procedure to the wrong patient
Retention of a foreign object in a patient following surgery or other invasive procedure
Any incident where the patient receives the wrong gas or oxygen through a line designated for a different gas or receives a toxic substance through a gas line
Any situation where care is ordered or provided by an individual impersonating a physician, nurse, pharmacist, or other licensed health-care provider
Abduction of a patient of any age
Sexual assault of a patient in or on the grounds of a health care provider
Artificial insemination with the wrong sperm or egg
Death during or immediately following surgery of a Class 1 patient
Death or serious injury of a patient by using a contaminated device, drugs, or biologics
Death or serious injury of a patient by using a medical device other than what the device was intended to be used
Death or serious injury of a patient due to an intravascular air embolism
Infant discharged with the wrong person
Death or serious injury of a patient due to the patient eloping from the medical facility
Death or serious injury of a patient who commits or attempts to commit suicide while in the care of a health-care facility
Death or serious injury of a patient due to a medication error
Death or serious injury of a patient due to receiving the wrong blood product type
Death or serious injury of a patient being cared for in a health-care facility for a low-risk pregnancy
Death or serious injury of a patient being cared for in a health-care facility at the time of a hypoglycemic episode
Death or serious injury of a neonate due to the failure to identify and treat hyperbilirubinemia
Death or serious injury of a patient following spinal manipulative therapy
Death or serious injury of a patient following electric shock or electrical cardioversion while in the health-care facility
Death or serious injury to a patient due to a burn from any source while a patient in the health-care facility
Death or serious injury to a patient due to a fall while a patient in the health-care facility
Death or serious injury of a patient due to the use of restraints or side rails while a patient in the health-care facility
Death or serious injury of a patient due to a physical assault in or on the grounds of a health care provider (Agency for Healthcare Research and Quality, 2017)

4.7.3   Value-Based Programs

Value-based programs are incentive programs providing additional payment to health-care providers who meet specific criteria based on the quality care they provide to their patients. These types of programs are intended to bring about change in health care with the focus on quality care while reducing overall cost (Centers for Medicare and Medicaid Services, 2017a). There are currently seven value-based purchasing programs. Table 4.2 provides information regarding six of the seven incentive programs not associated with long-term care. These incentive programs are worth reviewing for all of us. The potential exists for any one or more of these programs to become a value-based program in long-term care.

Table 4.2 Incentive programs for hospitals and home health

Value-based program	Program incentive	Program objectives	Program measures
Hospital Value-Based Purchasing (HVBP) Program	This program provides additional payment to hospitals for the quality care provided to Medicare patients	This is based on the hospital's ability to reduce adverse events, adopting evidence-based protocols, improving the care experience of patients, and reducing costs to Medicare	A variety of measures are used to determine when a hospital achieves the required outcomes including mortality, infection rates, safety, patient positive experience, and cost reduction (Centers for Medicare and Medicaid Services, 2017b)
Hospital Readmission Reduction (HRR) Program	This program links Medicare payments to the care received by Medicare recipients	The goal of this program is to reduce hospital readmission rates of Medicare recipients within 30 days of discharge with the same diagnosis	Important steps to take include coordinating care with receiving facilities or ensuring there are home services to meet the needs of the discharging patient, improved education to patients at the time of discharge so that they understand the steps they can take to improve their own outcomes, and sharing information with providers that is beneficial to the patient (Centers for Medicare and Medicaid Services, 2017c)
The Value Modifier Program	This program is based on the care provided by a physician and measures Medicare patient outcomes and cost	The modifier determines the reimbursement the physician will receive (Centers for Medicare and Medicaid Services, 2017d)	
Hospital-Acquired Condition Reduction Program	This program is intended to encourage hospitals to improve patient safety and reduce hospital-acquired conditions	Conditions include central line-associated bloodstream infection (CLABSI), catheter-associated urinary tract infection (CAUTI), surgical site infection, methicillin-resistant *Staphylococcus aureus* (MRSA), and clostridium difficile (C.diff)	Hospitals who are not able to improve safety or reduce the infections listed receive a reduced reimbursement rate, while hospitals that improve their scores receive a higher reimbursement rate (Centers for Medicare and Medicaid Services, 2017e)

(continued)

Table 4.2 (continued)

Value-based program	Program incentive	Program objectives	Program measures
End-Stage Renal Disease Program	This program is for out-patient dialysis units caring for Medicare recipients with end-stage renal disease	The goal is to improve outcomes in order to receive a higher reimbursement rate (Centers for Medicare and Medicaid Services, 2017f)	
The Home Health Value-Based Purchasing (HHVBP) Model	This program is intended for home health agencies providing care to Medicare recipients	This program is intended to provide financial incentives for home health agencies giving higher-quality care and more efficient care based on their outcomes	This program was rolled out in nine states in January 2016 (Centers for Medicare and Medicaid Services, 2017h)

There are several incentive programs identified for skilled nursing facilities.

4.8   Skilled Nursing Facility Value-Based Purchasing Program (SNFVBP)

This is a skilled nursing facility program that rewards nursing homes for quality care measures related to the care of Medicare recipients. However, this program has not officially started but is anticipated to begin in 2019. While the program has not officially begun, nursing homes are currently receiving quarterly feedback reports on their specific quality measures (Centers for Medicare and Medicaid Services, 2017g).

4.9   Pay for Performance

Pay for performance is an incentive program developed to give providers a financial incentive to meet and/or exceed specific quality requirements. Providers include physicians, hospitals, and nursing homes. Currently over half of Medicaid programs have some type of incentive program under pay for performance. Many of the programs have proven to show moderate success in following through on initiatives to improve the patient experience. Program goals include more efficient management of resources, promoting medical practices that provide a safe environment for patients, and following evidence-based practice in the provision of care (HealthAffairs 2012). Financial incentives may include any or all of the following outcome measures:

- Deficiency free survey
- Resident satisfaction
- Family satisfaction
- Employee satisfaction

- Continuing education of staff
- Nursing retention
- Nursing assistant retention
- Wound management
- Restraints
- Pain management
- Administration costs
- Operating costs
- Occupancy rates
- Person centered care
- Quality improvement
- Safety (Briesacher et al. 2009)

4.10   Private Insurance Controls: More Control Over Cost of Care

The health insurance industry grew out of a small service industry into a major third-party payer. With the economic downturn, employees are expected to shoulder more of the costs associated with their health care through increased co-payments and deductibles. Initially, the goal of requiring employees to pay for part of their health care was to help shoulder the burden of the rising cost of health care. The added goal is providing an incentive for employees to establish a healthier lifestyle in order to reduce health-care costs. Health insurers negotiate with providers to determine the rates that will be paid for care provided to health insurance consumers who carry the specific health insurance either through their employer or a private health insurance company.

With the inception of the Affordable Care Act, insurance companies are no longer able to refuse coverage based on pre-existing conditions. There are controls placed to reduce health insurance premium costs in states that are part of the health-care exchange. Despite these restrictions, we are still hearing stories regarding individuals who are not able to pay for health-care coverage and are forced to forgo the insurance knowing they face a penalty for not being covered. As the government considers the Affordable Care Act, there are many more questions regarding the future of health-care coverage across the United States. This will come to the forefront in 2018 and 2019 as the government determines the final outcome of the Affordable Care Act.

4.11   The Role of the LPN in Relationship to Fiscal Management Related to Billing and Coding

Overall the LPN does not have responsibility for billing and payment of services provided. Understanding how this works is beneficial to all nurses including LPNs. The goal is to maximize reimbursement within the guidelines provided through the prospective payment system developed by the Centers for Medicare and Medicaid

Services. When an older adult is admitted to a nursing home, the resident is identified with specific concerns related to the admission. For example, if your nursing home has a rehabilitation unit, the older adult might be admitted because they had a knee replacement. The primary diagnosis would be related to the knee replacement, and a code is generated identifying why the individual was admitted. If the older adult has other issues such as diabetes or high blood pressure, these issues would also be identified with a specific code, which is added to the older adult's record.

When the older adult (or anyone admitted to the nursing home) is admitted, a permanent record is generated that includes the diagnoses and codes identifying why the individual was admitted to the nursing home. The care team including nursing, therapy (if ordered), social services, dietary, and activities are required to document their admission assessments and any other services provided at the time of admission. Each professional providing care to the resident documents the care provided in the progress notes (nurse's notes) for each resident. This documentation is used by the individual completing the Minimum Data Set (MDS) to answer all the required questions. If there is something that cannot be answered, the individual completing the MDS can ask members of the care team to assist with answering the questions.

Each month the diagnoses and codes are used to bill the payer source for the services provided by the nursing home team. This information is included in each resident's permanent record and is accessed by the person who completes the billing through the Minimum Data Set (MDS) completed by the care team members. If there are errors in the billing process or the documentation required by the interdisciplinary team; reimbursement can be delayed, reduced, or denied. If reimbursement is reduced or denied; the organization will have more difficulty paying debts and providing the quality care expected. The close connection between accurate documentation related to the admission diagnoses as well as other diagnoses and reimbursement cannot be denied.

4.12   Review the Role of the Licensed Practical Nurse (LPN) Related to Appropriate Documentation of Patient Care

The LPN plays a critical role in the reimbursement process through appropriate documentation. When a new resident is admitted, your responsibility is to understand why the resident was admitted and to make sure your documentation reflects the rationale for admission as well as other diagnoses that impact the resident's daily life. For example, if a resident is admitted to the rehabilitation unit due to a fractured hip, your documentation needs to include information regarding the fractured hip and its impact on the resident. Questions you might consider include the following:

• Is the resident in pain? Where is the pain located? What is the level of pain intensity? What helps the pain? What makes the pain worse? How often is the resident taking pain medication?

- Is the resident able to participate in rehabilitation? If the answer is yes, therapy needs to be documented as well. You need to document how often the resident participates in therapy and the outcome of the therapy sessions.
- Is the resident able to complete ADLs with or without assistance? If the resident has limited ability to complete ADLs independently, it is important to document any limitations. By doing this, you will be able to track the resident's ability to complete ADLs and show improvement, no change in ability, or a decline in ability to complete ADLs.
- Is the resident able to ambulate? If not, what mobility aids or support does the resident use to move from one location to another? If yes, how far is the resident able to ambulate? Does the resident require assistance to transfer from one surface to another? If yes, what type of support does the resident need to transfer? Is the resident able to change position while in bed or in a chair. If not, what support does the resident need to change position while in bed? What support does the resident need to change position while in a chair?

Asking questions related to each diagnosis impacting the resident is important in order to provide complete documentation regarding the resident's current status, decline or improvement, and future goals based on the resident's plan of care. The LPN also has a responsibility of understanding the MDS process and the link between the MDS and documentation. If the documentation is not accurate, the MDS will not be accurate. If the MDS is not accurate, the RUGs' score will not be accurate. If the RUGs' score is not accurate, the reimbursement will not be accurate. In order to maximize reimbursement, the documentation needs to be accurate. This is an important role the LPN takes on as part of being a nurse in the long-term care setting. There is no substitute for accurate documentation.

References

Agency for Healthcare Research and Quality (2017) Never events. Retrieved from https://psnet. ahrq.gov/primers/primer/3

Briesacher B, Field T, Baril J, Gurwitz J (2009) Pay-for-performance in nursing homes. Health Care Financ Rev 30(3):1–13

Centers for Medicare and Medicaid (2008) Medicare and Medicaid move aggressively to encourage greater patient safety in hospitals and reduce never events. Retrieved from https://www.cms.gov/Newsroom/MediaReleaseDatabase/Press-Releases/2008-Press-Releases-Items/2008-07-313.html

Centers for Medicare and Medicaid (2015) NHE fact sheet. Retrieved from https://www.cms.gov/Research-Statistics-Data-and-Systems/Statistics-Trends-and-Reports/NationalHealthExpendData/NHE-Fact-Sheet.html

Centers for Medicare and Medicaid (2017a) What are the value-based programs?. Retrieved from https://www.cms.gov/Medicare/Quality-Initiatives-Patient-Assessment-Instruments/Value-Based-Programs/Value-Based-Programs.html

Centers for Medicare and Medicaid (2017b) The hospital value-based purchasing (VBP) program. Retrieved from https://www.cms.gov/Medicare/Quality-Initiatives-Patient-Assessment-Instruments/Value-Based-Programs/HVBP/Hospital-Value-Based-Purchasing.html

Centers for Medicare and Medicaid (2017c) The hospital readmissions reduction (HRR) program. Retrieved from https://www.cms.gov/Medicare/Quality-Initiatives-Patient-Assessment-Instruments/Value-Based-Programs/HRRP/Hospital-Readmission-Reduction-Program.html

Centers for Medicare and Medicaid (2017d) The value modifier (VM) program. Retrieved from https://www.cms.gov/Medicare/Quality-Initiatives-Patient-Assessment-Instruments/Value-Based-Programs/VMP/Value-Modifier-VM-or-PVBM.html

Centers for Medicare and Medicaid (2017e) Hospital-acquired condition (HAC) reduction program. Retrieved from https://www.cms.gov/Medicare/Quality-Initiatives-Patient-Assessment-Instruments/Value-Based-Programs/HAC/Hospital-Acquired-Conditions.html

Centers for Medicare and Medicaid (2017f) End-stage renal disease (ESRD) quality incentive program (QIP). Retrieved from https://www.cms.gov/Medicare/Quality-Initiatives-Patient-Assessment-Instruments/Value-Based-Programs/Other-VBPs/ESRD-QIP.html

Centers for Medicare and Medicaid (2017g) The skilled nursing facility value-based purchasing program (SNFVBP). Retrieved from https://www.cms.gov/Medicare/Quality-Initiatives-Patient-Assessment-Instruments/Value-Based-Programs/Other-VBPs/SNF-VBP.html

Centers for Medicare and Medicaid (2017h) The home health value-based purchasing (HHVBP) model. Retrieved from https://www.cms.gov/Medicare/Quality-Initiatives-Patient-Assessment-Instruments/Value-Based-Programs/Other-VBPs/HHVBP.html

HealthAffairs (2012) Pay-for-performance. Retrieved from http://www.healthaffairs.org/health-policybriefs/brief.php?brief_id=78

Medicaid.gov (2017) Keeping America healthy. Retrieved from https://www.medicaid.gov/

Medicare.gov (2017) The official U.S. government site for Medicare. Retrieved from https://www.medicare.gov/

U.S. Department of Health and Human Services (2017) Indian health service. The federal health program for American Indians and Alaska Natives. Retrieved from https://www.ihs.gov/

U.S. Department of the Interior (2017) Indian affairs. Retrieved from https://www.bia.gov/index.htm

U.S. Department of Veterans Affairs (2017) Access and quality in VA health. Retrieved from http://www.accesstocare.va.gov/

The Role of the LPN as a Leader and Manager in the Health-Care Setting

5

5.1 Description

This chapter provides a comparison of the leader and the manager in the health-care setting as well as how the LPN fits into each of these roles. A variety of leadership styles will be discussed in the context of the health-care environment and specific traits that define each style and how the LPN fits within the context of one or more leadership styles. The role of the manager will be explored using Patricia Benner's novice to expert nursing theory.

5.2 Objectives

1. Compare and contrast the role of leadership and management in the health-care setting.
2. Explain the role of the LPN as a leader.
3. Explain the role of the LPN as a manager.
4. Develop leadership skills to enhance their role as team leader.
5. Transformational leader in the development of person-centered care.
6. Transactional leader reinforcing culture change.
7. Developing a leadership style.
8. Reviewing the role of the manager based on Benner's novice to expert theory.

5.3 Compare and Contrast the Role of Leadership and Management in the Health-Care Setting

The terms leader and manager have been interchanged in the workplace. The two terms are very different in terms of the traits associated with leaders and managers. Table 5.1 provides terms used to describe leaders and managers (Arruda, 2017;

© Springer International Publishing AG 2018
C. Kruschke, *Leadership Skills for Licensed Practical Nurses Working with the Aging Population*, https://doi.org/10.1007/978-3-319-69862-5_5

Table 5.1 Leadership and Management Traits

Leaders	Managers
Visionary	Develops goals
Change agent	Maintain the status quo
Individual thinker	Thinks the same as other managers
Risk taker	Avoids risk
Long-term strategist	Short-term goals
Builds relationships	Prefers structure and systems
Coach people	Manage people
Innovative	Problem solver
Sense of self	Persistent
Self-made	Tough-minded
Dedicated	Hardworking
Intelligent	Intelligent
Leads	Hierarchical
Focus on organization as a whole	Day-to-day operations
Fearless	Enforcer
Not a manager	Can be a leader

Management Study Guide, 2017). Consider your role as a LPN, which traits describe you as leader and manager?

5.3.1   Leaders

Leaders have consistently been defined as those individuals at the top of the chain of command. In health care, such as positions are chief executive officer, chief financial officer, chief nursing officer, and the nursing home administrator or executive are considered leadership positions.

You need to consider the traits of a leader within the health-care environment and how these traits apply to you as an LPN. A leader is someone who motivates and inspires others to be their best selves. Consider how you can motivate a CNA to provide care to the residents in their charge. Motivation and inspiration takes many forms as you lead your team in the provision of quality care for the elders in your charge. You need to show your team your expectations by modeling the behavior you expect from them. Each day you arrive at work, you are able to choose the attitude you will reflect to your team. If you come to work in a bad mood, this mood will be shared by your team. Likewise, if you choose to be in a good mood, this mood will also be shared by your team. As the team leader for your unit or department, you need to motivate and inspire your team through your words and actions. Allow your team members to do the work they were trained to do by delegating these tasks and assignments to those who are trained to complete those tasks and assignments. Then, trust them to complete the delegated tasks. Check back with them from time to time to ensure they have the tools they need to complete the delegated tasks and assignments. Delegation allows your team members to grow, which positively impacts the entire team and increases their ability to provide the quality care expected. Remember the adage, "how you treat your employees is how they will treat the elders they care for." Leadership is not dictatorship but a covenant to treat your employees with respect and support their ability to grow within their roles. In addition, you need to remain grounded and realize your role as a leader is a gift based on those who are willing to follow you based on your willingness to lead with compassion and caring.

A leader focuses on the strategic plan. The LPN as a leader needs to know the goals and objectives associated with the strategic plan of the organization in order to lead effectively. Leaders need to be aware of the direction the organization is moving in so that each leader can bring his/her knowledge, skills, and abilities to fulfill the strategic plan. This includes the LPN. We have the capacity to make appropriate decisions improving the quality of care based on the strategic plan (Sun, 2017; Zaleznik, 2017).

Leaders have a vision of the future (Sun, 2017; Zaleznik, 2017). This requires us to look forward and be willing to take the necessary steps to ensure there is a future for the organization as well as our team members. The LPN is part of the future vision. As a LPN, I kept a vision of the future by continually learning as much as I could about the elderly I cared for, the staff I worked with, and the strategic plan of the organization. Gaining this information provided the clarity I need to look to the future and make sure I was forward-thinking. Part of this process is looking back at where we have been in order to seek the future. We need to avoid becoming complacent, willing to accept the status quo. We have to be willing to change and grow as leaders. This includes continuing education, even if we are not required to complete continuing education. Many states do not require nurses to obtain CEUs. Regardless, I challenge each of you to seek out education for your own edification. We can only grow as nurses when we are willing to reach out and learn. These actions of improving ourselves and embracing change help in becoming a transformational leader. The ability to inspire and motivate is a trait of a transformational leader (Cherry 2017).

Leaders need to understand emotional intelligence. We need to understand ourselves and our emotions so that we can lead with our minds instead of our emotions (Psychology Today 2017). We have to be aware of how we feel throughout the day so that we can keep our feelings in check, which in turn allows us to help others to keep their emotions in check. As I stated previously, we are able to choose how we are going to feel when we get up in the morning. We can be upset or we can be calm. Regardless of what is happening around us, we have this capacity. This is especially important for leaders. If we are not able to keep our own emotions in check, we will not be able to assist our staff when their emotions get the best of them (Goleman 2016).

Think about a situation where you had to keep your feelings in check and what that felt like. Now think about a time when you were not able to keep your feelings in check and what that felt like. When we lose control of ourselves, we tend to lose control of any situation we are in at the time.

The ability to affect change is limited when we are not able to keep our emotions in check. This concept is important for all leaders including the LPN. There may be times when you feel the only way to make your point heard is to allow your emotions to take over for you. However, this will not work because others will do the same and you will not be able to lead any changes necessary. In essence, you need to be the leader who does the right thing and maintains control of situations where emotions can get the best of those involved.

Think about a leader who you remember as being successful. What are the traits that leader possessed? Do you have any of those traits? When we consider ourselves in comparison to someone who is a good leader, we often downplay our own skills as a leader, deferring to that individual as an expert leader. However, if we really take the time to reflect on our own skills, we may find that we have at least one trait that is similar to the leader we admire the most. We need to realize that being a leader is not about being in charge, it is about understanding what needs to be done and sharing that information with others without the use of threats or intimidation. Rather, we use communication and information to influence others to complete the work that needs to be done (Ellis and Abbott 2013). We now need to consider leadership styles impacting all of us.

5.3.1.1 Leadership Styles Introduced Over the Years

There are a variety of leadership styles that have been introduced over the years. You may or may not have seen one or more of these leadership styles emulated by a leader in your current organization or another organization. While the leadership styles being discussed here are not an all-inclusive list, they do provide a basis for understanding how a leader might respond to a given situation. The point here is leaders can change their styles depending on the situation. While it is beneficial for you to understand these leadership styles, we have come to a crossroad in long-term care, and we need to move beyond the leadership styles identified here to styles that are more conducive to change. Review the following paragraphs that describe the leadership styles of the past and present. Think about previous leaders you have had in the past and current leaders. Do any of the leaders you are thinking about match any of the styles identified below?

The **autocratic leadership style** is based on the leader who needs to make a decision immediately or if the team has lost their focus and needs a more controlled leadership style to move forward (Ellis and Abbott 2013). For example, if a state survey results in deficiencies, you may need to be more direct explaining to your care team what needs to be done to correct each deficiency. This might include continuing education as well as changes in protocols. To make the necessary changes as quickly as possible, you may use an autocratic leadership style where you direct your team toward the changes that have to be made. While this is not the most effective leadership style as a long-term approach, used sparingly for short-term issues, this approach is able to meet specific emergent challenges and emergencies quickly. This leadership style requires you to be more direct with your team, providing specific outcome requirements and the steps to achieve those requirements. You also need to follow through and check back with the team to make sure the required changes were made using the steps provided. I recommend you switch leadership styles as quickly as possible once the changes are made and listen to your team when it is time for them to provide feedback regarding any changes made.

The **persuasive leadership style** is intended to be used when decisions are made by senior leadership within your organization. When this occurs, you need to persuade your team to implement the change without actually having input into the change (Ellis and Abbott 2013). The assumption must be made that the decision to implement the change was made by those in leadership who understand why the change needs to be made. In long-term care, I have had to persuade team members to make a change that was necessary. This required me to be honest and open regarding why the change had to be made and why I was requesting the change without input from the staff. This would take place if there was a survey and we received a deficiency. The leadership team would review the deficiency and determine the best approach to bring us back into compliance as quickly as possible. We would review the evidence regarding the issue and use the deficiency comments and evidence found to formulate the plan of correction. We would implement the plan immediately to ensure we were in compliance. While we used persuasion, we also used the autocratic style as discussed previously. This particular combination was useful in the circumstances where compliance had to occur as quickly as possible.

The **consultative style or collaborative style** is when the leader knows what decision needs to be made but is open to suggestions of team members (Ellis and Abbott 2013). In this case, if we have a recommendation from the survey team to make a change in a process but it is not considered a deficiency because what we have been doing is "acceptable," the leadership team will still review the recommendation and review the evidence regarding best practice. This is not a situation requiring immediate action. I would bring the recommendation and evidence to the team and ask for input regarding the best approach to implement the change necessary. This allows for the team to become part of the process rather than being told what is going to happen. While I might not be able to accept every recommendation, I would make sure to provide feedback regarding all recommendations made. We need to remember that this leadership style is more team-focused but still provides a level of "control" by the leader.

The **participative leadership style** provides the most team-based approach to making decisions regarding the changes that need to be made (Ellis and Abbott 2013). This is one of the management styles I have used most extensively in my role as a leader in the health-care setting. When using this style, I would determine a process or protocol that needs to be updated. I would bring the team together and ask for the team's input regarding the anticipated change. If the team was in agreement with the change needing to take place; I would defer the change to the team to research, develop, and implement. While I would check back with the team to make sure they had all the resources they needed, I would not interfere with their work. However, I would make myself available if the team members had any questions or concerns. This was my opportunity to mentor the team without telling them what to do. This style was effective in sending a clear message to the team that I believed in their knowledge, skills, and abilities to make this change effectively.

There is one more leadership style I would like to discuss here, and that is **the laissez-faire leadership style**. This is a style that describes the leader who is "hands-off." This leader delegates responsibility to his/her team members and then takes a "hands-off" approach. In this case, the leader does not provide any guidance related to the tasks delegated to the team. This leader may or may not provide the resources needed to make any changes necessary. While the team members may come together to resolve any issues on their own, they may not feel empowered but abandoned.

5.3.1.2 Leadership Styles Present and Future

There are a few leadership styles that have the potential to take us into the future as we embrace a culture change approach to long-term care that focuses on patient-centered care and patient-directed care. Review these styles and determine if you have known or know a leader today who exhibits any of these styles.

The **transactional leadership style** evokes images of several of the past leadership styles you read about in this chapter with a focus on current operational needs. This leader is concerned with the day-to-day operations of the organization and ensuring that all financial benchmarks are met. This leader uses praise and punishment to maintain the organization. The praise is in the form of incentives to "encourage" their employees to perform as required. This leadership style is used to improve overall performance of an organization and to ensure that the employees working for the organization "buy in" to the organization's immediate goals (allnurses 2012). This style of leadership might be used in situations where the nursing home is under scrutiny during a survey that has resulted in deficiencies and the need to move the organization back into compliance. This style is reminiscent of the autocratic leadership style.

The **transformational leadership style** emphasizes the importance of commitment through motivating employees to do their best work (allnurses 2012). This leader learns as much as possible about the strengths and weaknesses of each employee and matches employees to tasks based on the employee's strengths. This leader also mentors employees to turn weaknesses into strengths. This leadership style emphasizes proactively solving problems through a team approach rather than waiting for the problem to result in negative outcomes. This leader uses "management by walking around" to learn more about his/her team members by getting out of his/her office and interacting with staff as well as residents. This approach provides the opportunity to be a team member rather than a voice from above that dictates change rather than encouraging staff to be transformational leaders within their own positions.

The **person-centered leadership style** is an emerging leadership style that focuses on the individual rather than the institutional styles you learned about here. This leader considers each individual as being important to the present and future of the long-term care home, wherever that home may be and whatever that home looks like. This leader maintains the highest level of communication possible to ensure his/her team members have the knowledge needed to do their best for their residents and each other. Motivation is a key element as the person-centered leader motivates his/her team members through high expectations and growth rather than dictating and punishment (Fox 2017).

5.4   The Role of the LPN as a Leader

Consider your role as a LPN in the long-term care setting. You are working on a unit as the unit nurse. You have a team of certified nursing assistants (CNAs) working with you; the decision is made to change the staffing structure of the unit based on the needs of the older adults living on the unit. You need to communicate the changes to the CNAs and provide the leadership needed to make the changes. You have the option of telling them what the changes will be and make the changes or you can explain the situation and ask for the input of the CNAs in order to determine the best course of action to make the necessary changes. Consider what we have discussed regarding the role of the leader. Based on what you have read and your understanding of the needs of the CNAs who are part of your team, the best course of action is to work with your CNAs to determine how you can make the changes needed. In this way, the CNAs will be part of the solution and feel that their concerns are heard. In addition, you inspire rather than dictate, which is critical to the role of the leader.

5.4.1   Managers

Managers have been defined as those individuals at the mid-level range of the chain of command. These are the individuals who manage departments or units and have both leaders to report to and individuals who report to them. LPNs are leaders and managers based on the role they are playing at any given time. Characteristics of managers vary from the characteristics of a leader within the health-care environment.

A major focus of managers is managing people and the tasks they need to complete (Sun, 2017; Zaleznik, 2017). As we discussed previously, delegation is a key role you play as a LPN. You need to delegate appropriate tasks to care providers including personal care assistants and certified nursing assistants. You may also be in the role of a lead LPN with the added responsibility of delegating to other LPNs. When we delegate, we need to make sure the individual we delegate a task to has the ability to complete that task within his/her own scope of practice. Each of us who have a license or a certification must know our own scope of practice and adhere to it. In addition, when you are the person who delegates tasks to others, you have a responsibility to know that person has the knowledge, skills, and abilities to complete those tasks.

The manager focuses on the day-to-day operations within the organization. This means the managers look at the financial picture for the unit they are managing as well as the outcomes of the residents who live there (Sun, 2017; Zaleznik, 2017). This role requires the manager to be more controlling to meet the obligations associated with fiscal management and resident outcomes. This also coincides with the manager's focus on managing people. While the past relationship has been supervisor (manager) and subordinate, we have had a paradigm shift to team member with a blurring of the roles that is important in a culture change environment promoting human caring rather than tasks. Managers are detail-oriented in order to maintain their focus on operations. The style most associated with managers is the transactional style in order to promote structure.

Managers do not exhibit specific styles as defined for leaders. While we can associate the transactional leadership style as the style that best describes a manager within the context of his/her role, we need to consider what the manager does in order define a style of management. Patricia Benner's novice to expert nursing theory fits well when discussing the manager in his/her development of management skills and development of relationships over time (Nursing Theory 2016).

5.4.1.1 Novice Managers

When a nurse manager takes on the role of manager, he/she shifts back to a novice, based on Benner's novice to expert nursing theory. These managers have a steep learning curve especially if they are promoted from within and do not have any management experience. If the manager is new to the unit, getting to know the staff and residents will be critical to the manager's success. If the manager worked on the unit as a staff nurse, this manager will need to acclimate himself/herself as new manager and make the shift from peer to supervisor.

The ideal situation would be if the manager is provided with a mentor who can support the new manager as he/she increases his/her knowledge, skills, and abilities as a manager (Clark-Burg and Alliex 2017). However, as many of us know, many managers are promoted from staff nurse to nurse manager without a great deal of training in this new role. They may receive information regarding their job responsibilities, but, beyond education regarding their basic role, the balance of the information they need to learn is achieved through on-the-job training they provide themselves. Without a mentor, nurse managers are at risk to fail due to their lack of understanding regarding their new role. This is a very stressful period for a new manager because of his/her lack of understanding of the management role, his/her doubts regarding his/her own ability to manage, and his/her steep learning curve as described previously. This is the time when managers make the most mistakes and begin to doubt their own ability.

Without mentoring, many managers have failed in their new role and either shifted back to a staff nurse position or left the organization. I remember becoming a manager in a non-health-care setting. I was fortunate because I had already obtained my business degree and had a basic understanding of the role of a manager. In addition, I had been a LPN for 10 years and had the ability to apply my staff nurse knowledge, skills, and abilities to this new management role. I have also worked in organizations where staff nurses have been promoted to nurse manager and had difficulty acclimating to their new role because there was no formal orientation program. Some organizations provided some orientation, while others provided an orientation program as well as a mentor for the new nurse manager. The nurse managers who received formal orientation as well as a mentor were the most successful and had the highest retention rate. Those who had no training and no mentor were the least successful and had the lowest retention rate.

5.4.1.2 Advanced Beginner Managers

The advanced beginner has developed management skills. The manager who has support will move to the advanced beginner role much quicker than the manager who does not have support. This manager is making adequate decisions and building new management protocols that will help him/her to improve and grow in his/her role. In addition to building management skills, the advanced beginner manager is making strides to improve relationships with staff and residents. This is important for the manager who did not receive any formal training as a manager because more time was taken to develop management skills than building relationships. This manager is becoming more comfortable in the decision-making process.

I have witnessed managers at this level showing new skill at completing tasks assigned to them. They are more proficient in the day-to-day operations of the unit and have developed important relationships with staff and residents working and living on their unit. They are feeling more comfortable in their role but continue to seek guidance from their peers and leadership team. As a nursing home administrator, I made sure to mentor nurse managers to provide the support they needed to be successful. As a nurse manager at the advanced beginner stage, I did feel more confident completing the management tasks assigned to me. I was not ready to take on more tasks than those initially assigned to me. It became easier for me to get out of my office more to work with my team because I was able to complete required tasks more quickly. This was a sign to me I was learning and growing in my role, which made me more comfortable.

5.4.1.3 Competent Managers

When a new manager is able to learn his/her role and develop relationships with the residents and staff on the unit he/she manages, he/she moves from novice to advanced novice and then to a competent manager. This usually takes a minimum of 1 year but as long as 2–3 years to achieve. At this point in the managers' career, they have built a clear understanding of their role and the tasks they need to achieve. This manager has developed and nurtured his/her relationships with staff and residents who work and live on the unit.

The manager is now capable of having a voice in making unit and organizational changes. This manager thinks out of the box more often and sharing those ideas with the upper leadership team including the director of nursing and the nursing home administrator. While this manager has become more self-assured, continuing education and support remains critical to his/her success (Clark-Burg and Alliex 2017).

5.4.1.4 Proficient Managers

The proficient manager has more clarity regarding the role of manager and the steps necessary to make sound management decisions. With continued support, this manager is self-assured and continues to make more decisions with ease. This manager has developed more strategic relationships beyond those developed and nurtured on the unit. These relationships include interprofessional relationships both in the organization and outside the organization. The senior leadership team is able to delegate additional responsibility to this manager based on the manager's knowledge, skills, and abilities within appropriate limitations to avoid overwhelming the manager. This manager continues to make necessary changes and is able to share his/her knowledge regarding the changes made with other managers. Senior leadership needs to assist this manager in the development of his/her short-term and long-term goals for his/her professional growth.

5.4.1.5 Expert Managers

The expert manager no longer feels new in his/her management role. The manager is able to complete his/her tasks with ease and has a clear understanding of the policies, procedures, rules, and regulations that guide his/her management practice. They are able to make decisions using their understanding of management principles, their management intuition, and their nursing intuition. This manager is self-assured and is ready to mentor new managers regarding the management role (Clark-Burg and Alliex 2017).

As a nursing home administrator, this is the manager I relied on the most to assist with the decision-making process. This is also the manager I would delegate important tasks to because of his/her expertise and attention to detail. In addition, as the organization looks long term, this manager is in position to be considered for promotion. Mentoring this manager toward promotion is important both in terms of strategic planning and a means for continuing professional growth of this manager.

5.5   The Role of the LPN as a Manager

Your role as a LPN in the long-term care setting sets the stage for you to be a nurse manager for your specific unit. This is probably not a role you were trained to do as part of your education. While LPNs learn to be the right hand of the RN, becoming a nurse manager of a unit is not part of all LPN education. While the unit may have a manager overseeing all three shifts, the nurse manager is responsible for the shift he/she is working on. As a nurse manager, you are responsible for the unit when you are working. This means you need to be aware of the issues related to the residents and the staff and how these issues might impact other units or the organization. The CNAs working on your unit need to be aware of their responsibilities for the shift, which requires you to meet with them at the start of the shift and communicate your expectations for the shift. You also need to listen to the CNAs as they express their concerns for the shift that is beginning. While this reporting period is short, it is a strategic process ensuring your entire team is aware of the issues and you and your team have developed your plan of action for the remainder of the shift.

The most common issues faced by the nurse manager involve staff concerns, resident concerns, supply issues, and/or equipment issues. When faced with staffing concerns, involving the RN as quickly as possible is important. If your organization is large enough, involving the human resources department may also be prudent especially if the issue involves two or more CNAs with a difference of opinion. When it comes to resident concerns, you may need to involve the RN as well as other professionals such as the social worker or others depending on what the situation is. Here are several scenarios to work through:

- As a LPN working on a nursing unit, I had situations developed where one or more CNAs were not getting along. In some cases, the situation resolved itself, while in other cases, the CNAs were not able to resolve the problem and would come to me for assistance. It was critical to listen to each person involved and make sure he/she understood I was listening. During these conversations, you need to communicate clearly without taking sides. You need to allow each person the opportunity to explain his/her position and then repeat back to him/her what was said for clarification. Sometimes, allowing each person to express where he/she is coming from and how he/she feels is sufficient to resolve the issue. This is especially true when an individual just wants to be heard. There were times when we were not able to work through an issue immediately; I would then make an appointment with each person involved to discuss the situation further with the understanding the individuals involved would not discuss the issue further until they met with me. This was intended to avoid conflict between the initial discussion and when we could meet again. There were times the meeting itself helped with the resolution when each person heard how the other person felt, and by listening to how the other person felt, the individual could empathize and had better understanding of the situation which resulted in resolution. Your role as the nurse manager requires you to allow your team the opportunity to resolve issues on their own before you get involved. If they are unable to resolve the issue timely, you do need to assist them in any way you can before the conflict gets out of hand.
- Resident concerns are equally important to resolve. This includes concerns related to a resident and a staff member, a resident and another resident, and even a resident and a family member. This requires you to listen to what the residents are concerned about and ask them how they want the situation to be resolved. When you ask the residents how they want the situation resolved, they may state a resolution that cannot be met. For example, if residents are upset with the CNA caring for them, they may state they want the CNA terminated. This is not a possibility unless there is an accusation of some type and an investigation results in the CNA being terminated. Listening to the residents and validating their feelings and gaining their perspetive is critical. You also need to listen to the CNAs in question to determine their point of view regarding the issue. In these situations, involving the RN as soon as possible is critical. You may also need to involve other professionals such as the social worker if the problem is not able to be resolved.
- Staffing issues are very important to resolve as quickly as possible. As the nurse manager LPN, I avoided using the term "short staffed" due to the negative connotations associated with the term. The implication is that there is not enough

staff to provide care to the residents. I truly believe when we use a negative term, our viewpoint turns more negative. When we use the term "short staffed," the residents may hear this term and become very concerned that their needs are going to be met. In response to this fear, residents might use their call lights more often to obtain reassurance there was someone available to help them. You need to meet with the RN to discuss the staffing issue and determine the steps needing to be taken towards resolution. You should then meet with your team, explain the situation, and determine the resolution. For example, if one CNA calls in sick and there is no replacement, you need to work with the RN and your team to determine the best resolution. You might consider the following potential resolutions:

– Call in someone early from the night shift.
– Develop smaller work teams to ensure all residents have someone assigned to them.
– Ask the other units to send support throughout the shift. I have used this approach by having someone from another unit assigned to my unit for one hour at a time.

• Another area of concern is the issue of supplies and equipment. If you do not have sufficient or correct supplies or equipment available for resident care, you need to contact the RN immediately to assist you in resolving this issue. You may need to involve other professionals as the situation arises. For example, if you need a specific supply item or equipment and your organization has a supply person, you would contact that person to assist you in obtaining the supply item or equipment. You might also contact the other units to determine if they have the supplies or equipment you need. I have also had the experience of contacting our pharmacy to obtain a supply item such as wound dressings until our supplier could get the supplies to us. We have also contacted our supplier to overnight specific items needed. For equipment, if a resident needed a walker or wheelchair, we would ask the therapy department for the item. If the item is not available, the RN or central supply person can be contacted for assistance. In turn, the director of nursing can also be contacted to assist you to resolve the issue.

Regardless of the issue, the key is to resolve the issue as quickly as possible. This is your role as a nurse manager.

References

Allnurses.com (2012) Transactional leadership versus transformational leadership. Retrieved from http://allnurses.com/nurse-management/transactional-leadership-versus-759181.html

Arruda W (2017) 9 differences between being a leader and a manager. Retrieved from Forbes at https://www.forbes.com/sites/lizryan/2017/08/05/four-ways-youre-relinquishing-your-power-without-realizing-it/#f62ac0c609b6

Cherry K (2017) What is transformational leadership? A closer look at the effects of transformational leadership. Retrieved from https://www.verywell.com/what-is-transformational-leadership-2795313

Clark-Burg K, Alliex S (2017) A study of styles: how do nurse managers make decisions? Nurse Manag 48(7):44–49

Ellis P, Abbott J (2013) Leadership and management skills in health care. Br J Cardiac Nurs 8(2):96–99

Fox N (2017) Lessons in leadership for person-centered elder care. Health Professions Press, Baltimore, MD

Goleman D (2016) Women leaders get results: the data. Retrieved from http://www.danielgoleman.info/women-leaders-get-results-the-data/

Management Study Guide (2017) Leader versus manager. Retrieved from http://managementstudyguide.com/leader_versus_manager.htm

Nursing Theory (2016) Patricia Benner novice to expert: nursing theorist. Retrieved from http://nursing-theory.org/nursing-theorists/Patricia-Benner.php

Psychology Today (2017) Emotional intelligence. Retrieved from https://www.psychologytoday.com/basics/emotional-intelligence

Sun L (2017) Management vs. leadership. Retrieved from BusinessDictionary at http://www.businessdictionary.com/article/705/management-vs-leadership/

Zaleznik A (2017) Managers and leaders: are they different?. Retrieved from Harvard Business Review at https://hbr.org/2004/01/managers-and-leaders-are-they-different

Communication Skills for the LPN

6

6.1 Introduction

Communication is critical in the care of our patients and in the development of interprofessional and intra-professional relationships. Without excellent communication skills, we run the risk of making errors that can be detrimental to our patients and interfering with relationship and team building which are both critical to our health-care practice.

6.2 Objectives

1. Identify communication techniques.
2. Demonstrate understanding of interdisciplinary communication across the health-care continuum in relationship to the management of the care environment and the care of the older population.
3. Explore communication techniques to foster collaboration and team building.
4. Demonstrate understanding of therapeutic communication in relationship to the older population.

6.3 Communication Techniques

6.3.1 Formal

Our first step in understanding the communication process is to review the techniques we use in communicating.

Formal communication is the means we use to communicate formalized by our place of employment. For example, in many organizations, formal communication would include email, memos, and other forms of written communication. This type of communication is very important for your professional career.

© Springer International Publishing AG 2018
C. Kruschke, *Leadership Skills for Licensed Practical Nurses Working with the Aging Population*, https://doi.org/10.1007/978-3-319-69862-5_6

Consider the nursing home that uses email to communicate with their staff and provide updates. Even the shortest email would be considered formal communication because it is used in your organization. There are a variety of rules that have been developed to address how an email is written. I would like to share a few of those rules with you. These rules can be applied to any written communication.

- Keep the written communication as succinct as possible while maintaining the intent of the message.
- Read what you have written before you send the email or any form of written communication.
- Do not use email or any other form of written communication when you are angry. Take the time to reflect and calm down before communicating with anyone. You might consider speaking with the person you are upset with in person to resolve any issues.
- Make sure the subject line accurately depicts the content of the email.
- Start the email or memo with a brief description so that the reader knows what the primary content of the written communication is. This is also a means of reminding the reader regarding previous discussions or comments with the author of the email or memo.
- Use bullet points if you have more than one topic or question to pose.
- Avoid using bold print unless absolutely necessary.
- Do not use all capital letters to emphasize a word; this is considered "yelling" in an email or memo.
- Make sure the font is easy to read. Do not use arbitrary font such as "curlz mt" in 10 font. This would make the email or memo difficult to read especially for someone like myself who is a baby boomer. Be gentle on my eyes please.
- Avoid using reply all to emails unless absolutely necessary. Consider which recipients actually have to see your reply. There is nothing more disheartening than to have an important email or memo that has secure content sent to more individuals than those who really need to read the email or memo.
- If you are replying to an email that is attached to a string, read the entire string before responding.

6.3.2 Informal

Informal communication is usually used at home but can also be used in the workplace. Whether in a meeting or face-to-face verbal communication that is casual would be considered informal. In the workplace, this type of communication may occur during the following situation:

- Individuals meet casually to discuss work or personal situations.
- Prior to or after a more formal meeting.
- During phone conversations that may or may not include more formal communication.
- This type of communication may also be considered "gossip" or "grapevine banter."

6.3.3   Face-to-Face

When you are speaking to one or more individuals, plan to face the person you are speaking to. This includes the use of body language. When you face someone to speak with that person, you also need to turn your body in that same direction. Avoid crossing your arms, but keep them loosely at your side or resting on the table if you are sitting at a table or desk.

6.3.4   Technology

Technology in communication includes the technology we use in the communication process. This includes technology such as computers, emails, pagers, cell phones, text messages, social media, and apps. In addition, communication can be used to help individuals understand communication better such as translation lines, voice simulators, and speech assistive devices.

6.3.5   Verbal

Verbal communication refers to our ability to communicate using words. With each generation we become more diverse with a variety of languages spoken. This requires us to be more aware of the language our patients speak to ensure we provide the support needed to communicate with them.

6.3.6   Nonverbal

Nonverbal communication includes body language, gestures, facial expressions, posture, voice changes such as inflection and tone, physical touching, and physical space. A high percentage of communication is nonverbal in nature (thebalance, 2017; Green, 2013).

6.3.7   Listening

Effective communication includes effective listening skills. This requires you to actively listen to the other person. Ask questions to obtain clarification of what you heard. You also need to avoid formulating your response while the other person is still speaking. Good listening skills also mean you allow the other person to finish what they are saying before you begin speaking. You do not begin speaking while the other person is speaking. Part of good listening is to make sure you are not overspeaking the other individual. I use the term overspeaking when the listener jumps in and begins speaking before the other individual has finished speaking, resulting in both of you speaking at the same time.

6.4 Communication that Fosters Collaboration and Team Building

The ability to collaborate is tied to our ability to communicate. This is especially true for leaders. We need to communicate effectively in order to foster collaboration. If we do not bring clarity to our communication, we run the risk of having professionals we work with doubt what we are saying and stop listening. For you the LPN leader, you need to be honest and bring truth and clarity to everything you say. Previously, we discussed how management by walking around helps the leader or manager get to know the individuals they work with and the residents they care for. Excellent communication skills are the frontline of building a collaborative work environment where professionals you work with are ready to collaborate with you because of your ability to communicate the information necessary to sustain the collaborative atmosphere as well as an atmosphere fostering team building. When you are not clear with your communication, your ability to be collaborative or promote team building will be compromised.

6.5 Intra-professional Communication

Intra-professional communication takes place between professionals within the same facility (Thistlethwaite, 2015). For example, when a patient in the acute care setting is admitted first to the emergency department and then is transferred to the medical unit, the nurse from the emergency department will contact the nurse working on the medical unit to update the medical unit nurse regarding the patient being transferred. This is intra-professional communication.

Additional intra-professional communication taking place between members of the interdisciplinary team (Thistlethwaite, 2015). Includes the following examples:

- A nurse in the nursing home setting contacts the physician to obtain additional orders.
- The nurse informs the director of nursing that a care provider did not report to work as assigned.
- The RN completes the MDS and shares the revised care plan with the care team including the LPN and the CNAs on the unit.
- The LPN reports a fall to the RN, providing the data collected related to the fall.
- The RN or LPN delegates a care task to a CNA.
- The CNA reports to the nurse when a resident reports pain.

Communication takes place with each change of shift between the nurses and the nursing assistants:

- The nurse going off duty reports to the nurse coming on duty.
- A CNA going off duty may report a specific issue regarding a resident with a CNA who is coming on duty. The CNA coming on duty reports what is learned with the shift nurse.

- The nurse has received report from the previous shift nurse and now gives report to the CNAs.

Communication takes place between departments:

- A nurse contacts the internal pharmacy to deliver a newly ordered medication.
- The physical therapist provides an update to the nurse regarding a patient's therapy session and pain level.
- The physical therapist discharges a patient from therapy. The patient will now receive restorative therapy. The therapist explains the restorative therapy steps to the CNAs and nurses.
- A nurse contacts the maintenance department and speaks to the supervisor regarding a maintenance issue on the unit.
- A housekeeper notifies a member of maintenance to report a broken overbed table.

Communication is critical to the health-care environment. Think about the number of conversations you are part of in one shift. Would you be as successful without this level of communication?

6.6   Barriers to Communication Between Team Members

There are a variety of communication barriers impacting effective communication between team members. Each of us brings a variety of attributes to the communication process including our background, age, gender, and education to the process of communication. We need to understand barriers to communication impeding this process.

6.6.1   Upward and Downward Barriers to Communication

Upward and downward communication refers to the communication taking place between leaders and managers and their direct reports. For example, a licensed practical nurse (LPN) communicating with a certified nursing assistant (CNA) would be using downward communication. When the communication is reversed, the CNA would use upward communication to the LPN. This is not implying the LPN is better than the CNA; the implication is that the LPN is in a higher position than the CNA based on the organization reporting chart. There are a variety of variables that can impede upward and downward communication.

Differing communication skills can impede communication especially if one person has a higher level of communication skill in comparison to the other individual involved in a conversation. Think about the differences in communication style from a baby boomer to a millennial. The individual considered a baby boomer was raised writing letters and communicating in person, while the individual considered the millennial was raised using technology to communicate. If the millennial prefers to text, their ability to verbally communicate might reflect this approach. The same applies regarding educational level. As we move through the school system from elementary school to high school to the college level, our ability to communicate also changes. We develop a larger vocabulary and have more opportunity to communicate with others at or above our own level of communication. This is not to imply someone with an elementary school level of communication is not as intelligent as someone with a college education; it is the level of education coupled with experiences at or above that level that can shift our communication style. For example, I communicated differently before becoming a nurse and after becoming a nurse. Initially, my experiences were limited. But, as my experiences grew, so did my ability to communicate. I communicate differently today than I did 10 or 20 years ago due to education and experiences.

Fear is another factor that needs to be taken into consideration. When I first became a LPN and I spoke with my supervisors, I was very cautious regarding how I spoke with them and what I said to them. Part of this is a learned behavior watching how other individuals spoke with the supervisor. If someone is reprimanded for how they are speaking with their supervisor, you might not use that same approach. If someone is speaking with their supervisor and the supervisor is receptive to what is being said, you might consider that approach in the future. If I am afraid of my supervisor, I might avoid communicating with that individual as much as possible. This fear would impede my ability to communicate, which would be detrimental especially if there was information I needed to provide to my supervisor. For the leader, if you are communicating in such a way as to cause fear, you need to review your communication style. This is achieved by obtaining feedback from others regarding your communication style. The ability to "read" facial expressions will help you understand how others interpret what you are saying.

Position when communicating is another factor to consider. This is not referring to where you when communicating, but your position in the organization. We discussed upward and downward communication previously. This type of communication is based on position. When moving up the chain of command, you would have the movement depicted in Fig. 6.1 upward communication.

Downward communication is depicted in Fig. 6.2 downward communication.

6.6.2   Lateral Barriers to Communication

Lateral communication refers to communication between peers at the same level of the organization. This would include CNA to CNA, LPN to LPN, RN to RN, director to director, and administrator to administrator. See Fig. 6.3 Lateral Communication.

There are a variety of variables that can impede communication moving laterally. Many of these variables are the same as found in upward and downward communication. **Differing communication skills** is a variable that has the capacity to impede communication between individuals on the same level in the organization. While individuals at the same level within an organization might be assumed to have the

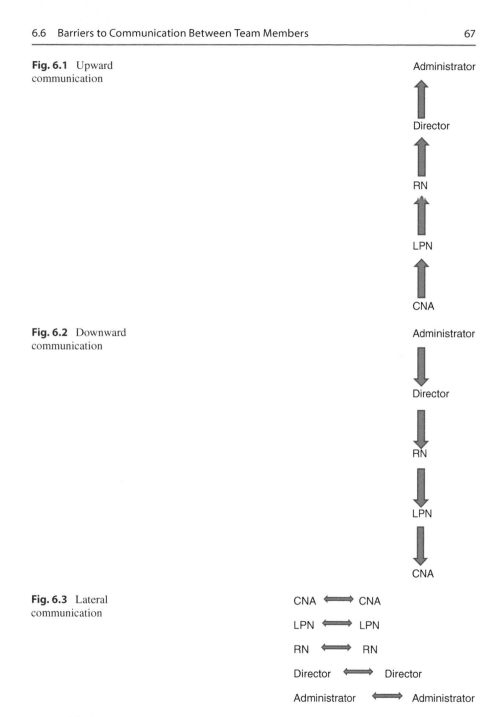

Fig. 6.1 Upward communication

Fig. 6.2 Downward communication

Fig. 6.3 Lateral communication

same skill level, this is not the case. Differences can occur including age, gender, and **education level** beyond the required education for a specific role.

   Fear can also occur when reviewing the barriers to lateral communication. This is not fear of a supervisor but fear of a peer who is on the same level. There may be a variety of reasons why we might fear a co-worker. It is possible we have a fear of communication in general or that the fear is actually embarrassment. We might also have a fear of a co-worker if that co-worker is not easy to communicate with. I have worked with individuals who have not been easy to communicate with. They have been confrontational and opinionated and not in a good way. They had hard opinions of others and were often critical. This is the type of person you might have heard someone refer to by saying "they have always been this way" or "that is just _____." When these statements were made, I often wondered how this person was allowed to be inconsiderate to others. Another type of fear is the fear of becoming involved in an argument. This can lead individuals to avoid open communication that might include a difference of opinion. This person is so fearful of confrontation of any level they are not willing to be open about opinions especially if their opinion was different from someone else. A third type of fear involves an individual who is afraid of "feeling less than" when speaking to a peer. This fear results in the individual not communicating with others to avoid having this feeling. I have worked with individuals who were afraid of speaking with others because of having this feeling. These individuals need encouragement to feel secure enough to voice their opinion.

Another obstacle associated with lateral communication is **familiarity** with the individual you are communicating with. If you do not have familiarity with the individual, communication may be limited until that person can build some type of working relationship with you. On the other hand, if you are friendly with the individual you are communicating with, you may speak to that person differently than you would someone you are less familiar with. We need to remember when you are communicating with someone in the workplace regarding the workplace, you need to elevate your communication to a more professional level than you would if you were speaking with this person outside the workplace. We have to be able to keep our professional and our personal lives separate when it comes to communication.

The **use of jargon** is an obstacle that is not always considered when speaking with an associate regardless of their level in the organization. Consider communicating with individuals from different departments. Each department and/or profession have their own jargon used to speak with each other. For example, as a nurse, you understand the terminology used by other nurses. However, when speaking with someone from therapy, you may not know all the jargon used by that department/profession. You should avoid using jargon specific to nursing to ensure a higher probability of being understood during the communication process. This is especially important when communicating with residents and/or family members.

When one or more individuals communicating have a **lack of interest** in the topic being discussed, it is much more difficult to communicate effectively. The other individual may not always listen to the entire conversation and thus miss part or all of the message being delivered. It is not always easy to determine when someone has lost interest. Consider the following signs as you communicate:

- Lack of focus on the conversation. As you communicate back and forth, the other individual does not respond to questions or make appropriate comments based on what you said.

- Easily distracted. Lack of eye contact. Requires you to repeat information already shared.

We cannot assume the individual is being distracted on purpose. Many individuals who become distracted may be very busy or distracted on a variety of issues. When you see someone is distracted, consider having the conversation at another time. You might also consider slowing down the conversation to make sure the individual does understand what you are saying, which will make it easier for that individual to engage in the conversation.

6.7 Differences Impacting Communication

6.7.1 Cultural

Despite our growing global society, there are cultural differences that can and will impact our ability to communicate with others. We are seeing more diversity in the workplace both from the perspective of the caregivers and also from the perspective of the residents/patients/clients we care for. We need to take into consideration that different cultures have differing "rules" that are followed in the process of communication. Consider the following:

- There are cultures where eye contact during the communication process should be avoided (Bright Hub Education, 2014).
- In one culture, the handshake is appropriate, whereas in other countries, the handshake is not appropriate (Cotton, 2013).
- In some cultures, proximity to the other individual while communicating is avoided, while other cultures allow for close proximity when communicating.
- Some cultures avoid confrontation even at the cost of personal opinion, while other cultures embrace confrontation as a means to express oneself and to come to agreement.
- Touching the head in some cultures is offensive, while in others, using the feet to point is offensive (Cotton, 2013).
- In some cultures, expressing pain is not done, while in other cultures, expressing pain is expected.
- Cultural differences also apply to who makes decisions for the care of a patient. In some cultures, the oldest male adult might make the decisions, while in another culture the patient makes their own decisions.
- In some cultures, having someone of the opposite sex provide hands-on care is not allowed, while in other cultures, female caregivers are expected (Gut et al. 2017).

As we become more global, we need to learn about the cultures of those we work with and provide care to. We may not be able to learn about every culture, but learning information regarding those we work with and care for makes a great deal of sense in order to build our communities within our own care environments.

The LPN has an important role in this process by learning about the cultures related to the aging population you are caring for as well as the cultures of those you work with. The first step is to read about each culture and learn the important "dos and don'ts." Sit down and talk to those you care for and work with to learn more about them and their culture. Listen attentively and ask questions to obtain additional information. Alter your approach to communication to meet the needs of the resident, family members, and other caregivers. Taking these initial steps will be beneficial in the long run as you become more knowledgeable about those you care for and those you work with.

6.7.2 Language

When we work with caregivers who speak another language and English is considered a second language, there are obstacles to the communication process that need to be considered. This also applies to residents/patients/clients who speak another language and English is considered a second language. When we travel to other countries, we attempt to adapt to a specific country by reading about the country and learning a few words to communicate in the language of that country. We are finding as we become more global that individuals in other countries also speak English on a variety of levels depending on the requirements of that country (Lemfuss, 2012).

We need to help our residents, family members, and members of our care teams to overcome obstacles associated with language. We know members of our care team need to speak and write English as part of their job requirements. Learning our language can be daunting because the English language is one of the most difficult languages to learn. Beyond the basic "rules" of the language are the nuances that take us beyond the rules of English. For example:

1. The use of slang terms can leave individuals from other cultures wondering what we mean. For example, the word "bad" can mean good depending on the context of its use. Blowing up your phone means many calls and texts, not the actual meaning of "blowing up." We might also "blow up" if we drink or eat a lot. Of course, we might also be binging out. See what I mean?
2. There are words that are spelled the same and sound the same but have different meanings. The term for this is a "homograph" (Dictionary.com, 2017). For example, the word back can mean you have returned or referencing the opposite of your front. Another example is the word "bat" which can mean the object you hit a ball with or the mammal. Here are a few more for you:

   - Bark
   - Box
   - Close
   - Dear
   - Desert
   - Duck
   - Foot
   - Jam

- Pitcher
- Rock
- Wound

Can you think of other examples of a homograph?

3. There are words that are spelled differently and sound the same but have different meanings. The term for this is a "homonym" (vocabulary.com, 2017). For example, the words "bow" and "bough" sound the same, are spelled differently, and have different meanings. Another example is "their," "there," and "they're." Here are a few more for you to consider:

- To, too, two
- Dye, die
- Pear, pair
- No, know

Can you think of other examples of a homonym? Those of us who learned English as children understand these nuances in our language. However, if English is a second language, individuals may not understand all nuances. It is up to us to help and guide individuals.

6.7.3   Perception

Differences in language can change our perceptions especially related to how we describe events. As we learned previously, words with different meanings change context of communication when these words are used. Understanding these words is critical to our ability to express our perceptions of the world around us. While there are studies indicating the English language is easy to learn, there are other studies indicating the English language is not easy to learn. Our ability to learn English as a second language will impact our perceptions of the world around us based on our ability to communicate with others. Our perceptions also impact our point of view related to the English language. Our point of view comes from our background and what we have learned throughout our life. Caring for others requires a high level of communication skills beyond knowing the basics of the English language.

6.8   Physical Barriers to Communication

6.8.1   Impaired Hearing

There are a variety of physical barriers that can impact communication. Impaired hearing impacts the ability to communication due to loss of hearing. If someone cannot hear what is being said, the possibility exists the individual with a hearing loss will miss part or all of a conversation. This hearing loss can be temporary or permanent. When an individual has a great deal of wax buildup in the ear, the hearing loss will subside once the ears are flushed. If the individual has nerve damage, the possibility is strong the individual will not hear part or all of the conversation. Caregivers need to assist the older adult to maintain adequate hearing by keeping the ears clean and making sure individuals have their hearing checked annually or as needed. You as the LPN should be checking the ears of your residents to ensure the inner ear is free of debris such as wax. Many of us know someone who is hard of hearing and wears a hearing aid. We also know individuals who are hard of hearing and refuse to wear a hearing aid. There are a variety of ways to assist residents with impaired hearing to communicate including:

- Hearing aid.
- Word board that has well-known words such as "food" or "meal" included which the resident can point to as an assistive device for communication.
- The use of a computer to type words is an appropriate form of technology to assist with communication.
- Good eye contact.
- Slow speech down enough that the individual who can read lips can do so.

6.8.2   Speech Issues

Speech issues can have a negative impact on the ability to communicate. Consider the resident who is living with the side effects of a stroke and is not able to speak clearly. This can be very disheartening and could result in the resident not being willing to communicate. When you care for a resident who is having difficulty with speaking, a referral to speech therapy would be important to obtain. This provides the resident with an interdisciplinary approach to this issue in order to resolve the speech issue or learn ways to overcome the speech issue. For example, if someone has had a stroke and is not able to speak clearly, having the interdisciplinary team work together with the resident to the appropriate communication tool(s) would be beneficial to the resident.

Many years ago, I had a resident who had had a stroke and was no longer able to speak except for one word "beautiful." We used word boards and good eye contact to communicate with the resident. The resident would say the word "beautiful" with deferring inflections to express how she was feeling. Over time, we were able to understand what the resident was trying to say.

Another resident had a stroke after living in our nursing home for several years. This individual was originally from Puerto Rico, and English was his second language. He was able to speak English until his stroke. After the stroke, he was no longer able to understand or speak English. We tried the language line but the resident did not like using as demonstrated by him shaking his head in the negative. We provided him with an interpreter as well as a language board that had common pictures such as food and a glass for him to point to. Above the picture was the Spanish word for each item, and below the picture was the English word for each item. The picture board was made by the resident's decision-maker based on the words the resident would understand and connect to specific pictures. Through the use of the language board and interpreter, we were able to develop a new relationship with the resident.

With both of these residents, I was the nurse (LPN) who worked the most with them, and through a collaborative relationship with the resident and decision-maker as well as other team members including the CNAs, we were able to develop a plan of communication to overcome the obstacles associated with these residents. Using these same techniques, we were able to help residents who had other obstacles to communication overcome those obstacles and develop new approaches to communication.

6.9   Nonverbal Communication

When we consider the process of communication, we also need to consider nonverbal communication. This includes body language and written communication. There are a variety of signals that can be sent through body language. Consider your facial expressions, gestures you use, your posture, eye contact and your overall appearance. Are you sending the message intended?

6.10   Interprofessional Communication

- Acute care
- Long term care
- Home health care

Regardless of the health-care setting, interprofessional communication is communication that takes place between professionals in two separate facilities (Thistlethwaite, 2015). For example, when a patient is transferred to the hospital emergency department from a nursing home the nurse from the nursing home will contact a nurse in the emergency department to report current information regarding the resident (patient) who was transferred.

Additional examples include the following:

- A nurse from the hospital contacts the admitting facility or home health agency to provide report on a patient who has just been discharged to that provider.
- The director of nursing from one nursing home contacts the director of nursing from another nursing home asking for a protocol for frequent falls.
- The home health nurse admitting a patient from the nursing home (hospital) contacts the discharging nurse to receive current information regarding the patient.

6.11   Strategies to Communication

Communication strategies can be formalized policies regarding the communication process or as simple as developing a personal strategy to improve your own communication skills. Regardless of the depth of the strategy, the goal should be to develop a communication plan that emphasizes the message that needs to be communicated and how to complete the communication process to effectively communicate the message.

The questions you need to consider include Who, What, Where, When, How, and Why:

- **Who** is the message for? Make sure the person you are speaking with is the correct person. For example, when discussing a patient, is the person you are speaking with entitled to receive information? If you are having difficulty, are you speaking to someone who can help you make a decision? If you need a decision, is the person you are speaking to the right person to make the decision?
- **What** is the message I am trying to convey? You need to think about the message before you send the message. Write it down and reflect on the message.
- **Where** should the communication take place? Are you in the correct location? Take into consideration the need for privacy.
- **When** should the communication take place? "Cooler heads prevail." Write the email and wait to send when emotions are involved.
- **Why** does that individual need to receive the message? Is this a crucial conversation? Is the message necessary?
- **How** will I deliver the message to be most effective? Is an email sufficient or would a verbal discussion convey the message more appropriately.

6.12   SBAR Communication

Situation-Background-Assessment-Recommendations (SBAR) is an excellent tool to communicate between health care practitioners when discussing patients. For the LPN working with the aging population, the use of SBAR provides an application tool used for conversations that occur related to the patient regardless of the setting. SBAR can be used to communicate between the LPN and physician, LPN to Registered Nurse (RN), LPN to LPN and LPN to Certified Nursing Assistant (CNA).

The elements of SBAR communication include the following:

S = Situation: The current situation of the patient (The Joint Commission, 2017; Institute for Healthcare Improvement, 2017). What has changed? What was observed versus what was told to you? When did this situation occur? What preceded the change and how is the patient doing now?

B = Background: What is the background of the patient (The Joint Commission, 2017; Institute for Healthcare Improvement, 2017). including admission date, date of change, current medications, current labs, and imaging. Include interview of patient and caregivers if possible. Current vital signs taken by the LPN, and advance directives and code status.

A = Assessment:Your assessment is actually the compilation of the data collection process.The information you collected and reported should speak for itself. LPNs do not complete assessments. Only the RN or physician is able to complete an assessment. Therefore, your assessment is the information you provide (The Joint Commission, 2017; Institute for Healthcare Improvement, 2017).

R = Recommendation: This is the point where you discuss the plan with the RN or physician. While you do not order anything, you can certainly make recommendations based on your own experience or at the request of the patient or the RN. For example, you may have discussed the issue with the RN and the RN recommends an Emergency Room visit. This can be relayed to the physician (The Joint Commission, 2017; Institute for Healthcare Improvement, 2017).

6.13 Communication Between Caregivers and Older Adults

- The next step in our discussion regarding communication will involve how we can ensure communication takes place between caregivers and elders we are providing care to. For our purposes, we will focus on communication between caregivers and elders. Communication with patients occurs when a professional discusses the needs of the patient directly with the patient. This form of communication requires a two-way conversation allowing the professional as well as the patient to participate in the communication process. Communication with family members can take place between the professional and family member; the professional, patient, and family member; or between the patient and the family member. In all cases, any discussion with the family member regarding a specific patient requires the approval of that patient. If the patient is not able to make their own decisions and has a guardian or an activated power of attorney, then the guardian or power of attorney must give permission for the professional to talk to any other family members.

6.14 Barriers to Communication Between Caregivers and Older Adults

Communication with patients occurs when a professional discusses the needs of the patient directly with the patient. This form of communication requires a two-way conversation allowing the professional as well as the patient to participate in the communication process.

Communication with family members can take place between the professional and family member; between the professional, patient, and family member; or between the patient and the family member. In all cases, any discussion with the family member regarding a specific patient requires the approval of that patient. If the patient is not able to make their own decisions and has a guardian or an activated power of attorney, then the guardian or power of attorney must give permission for the professional to talk to with any other family members.

6.14.1 Diversity and Communication

- Consider the background of the older adult when planning to communicate with your resident.
- You need to consider the age, sex, religion, cultural background, country of origin, successful acclimation or acclimation issues related to moving to this country, etc. We are all impacted by our backgrounds related to these and other variables.
- You need to understand the background of your resident even in general terms. For example, if you ask an older adult if he/she is in pain and they say no but he/she is obviously in pain, the individual's background may include the fact that in the culture of this patient, expressing pain is considered a weakness or remaining stoic an expectation.

View this YouTube Video: Elder Communication
http://www.youtube.com/watch?v=YFdwcXSBCX0
Professional to patient: Talking with the Elderly:
http://www.youtube.com/watch?v=ZDpPQGkuWo0

6.14.2 Confidentiality

Medical personnel are required to maintain patient confidentiality especially related to communication of the patient's medical information. The Health Insurance Portability and Accountability Act (HIPAA) was enacted to protect patient's personal and medical information. The patient must be consulted prior to revealing any medical or personal information to someone else including family members. Only those individuals designated by the patient are allowed to receive this type of information. If the patient is not able to make this decision, the guardian or activated power of attorney is able to make this decision for the patient. For example, if a decisional patient does not want his or her spouse or significant other know about their medical status, medical personnel are not allowed to share that information with the spouse or significant other. Always check the patient's chart for authorization before sharing the patient's information.

6.14.3 Therapeutic Techniques

Communication between the medical professional and the older adult patient needs to follow both adult learning theory and therapeutic communication techniques. The adult learning theory reminds us that adults prefer to learn about themselves through participation in the process. Past experiences impact the ability to understand concepts, which requires us to speak in "layman's terms" rather than using medical jargon. We also need to consider all forms of communication including verbal, nonverbal, and written communication. When communicating, consider the following:

- Your position while sitting or standing
- Your use of good eye contact
- The inflection of your voice
- The speed of your speech
- Your facial gestures

Remember, how you communicate with family, friends, and patients is different. In addition, communicating with an older adult is different from communicating with younger individuals related to the older adult's background and ability to comprehend the communication. Avoid colloquialisms when communicating which include slang terms, contractions, and profanity.

When communicating with the older adult, being an attentive participant in the conversation is necessary.

- Come down to the level of the older adult. Stand if they are standing. Sit if they are sitting or lying down.
- Use appropriate nonverbal communication skills: body relaxed, arms down, and relaxed, facing the resident.
- Lean toward the older adult
- Eye contact
- Attentive listening
- Clarify

6.14.4 Interviewing Techniques

- In order to communicate with the older adult, we need to make sure the older adult feels welcome to the conversation. This requires us to maintain eye contact at the level of the patient. If you are standing while the older adult is sitting, eye contact is difficult to maintain. Sit down and face the older adult.
- Use non-threatening language and gestures. Speak in a normal tone of voice unless you determine the patient is not able to hear what you are saying. Use simple but complete sentences. Avoid accusatory language. Ask open-ended questions that allow the patient to comment freely.
- Make sure the location of the conversation is private and free from distractions.

- Avoid medical jargon and colloquialisms. Speak at the level of the older adult.
- Listen and ask clarifying questions to make sure you understand what the older adult is saying. Avoid judging what the older adult is saying.
- End the conversation by reviewing what was discussed and the plan of action to be taken. Make sure to allow the older adult to share their understanding of the conversation and the plan of action to be taken.

6.14.5 Communication Barriers both Written and Oral

Understanding barriers to communication is an important element in the communication process. If barriers exist, communication may break down resulting in misunderstandings and errors in judgment or plan of action. While we may have discussed several of these barriers previously, they warrant listing here for your review:

- Poor listening skills.
- Distractions that interfere with communication.
- Using inappropriate or distracting verbal and nonverbal cues. For example, tapping your foot or rolling your eyes might convey to the older adult that you are bored or impatient. Crossing your legs away from the individual or crossing your arms.
- Trustworthy. For example, if you are not totally honest with the patient, or say two different things regarding the same topic, the older adult may find you to be untrustworthy. Above all, be honest. Telling a patient you are giving them candy, then giving them medication is not trustworthy or ethical.
- Impatience due to lack of time. For example, you need to be patient with the older adult and allow them enough time to express themselves regarding their needs.
- Environmental issues. If the environment is not conducive to a therapeutic conversation, find an alternative place and time to have a conversation. You need to consider the type of environment that is conducive to a therapeutic conversation in advance of the conversation. Plan ahead.
- Tone of voice. Avoid a harsh or accusatory tone or word choice. If you are in a bad mood, your mood will reveal itself in your tone of voice or inflection. Use "I" statements rather than "you" statements. Ask questions for clarification rather than assuming anything.
- Age bias. Consider your feelings and beliefs regarding the older adult. An older adult is not a big child. Wrinkles do not imply the individual cannot understand what you are saying. Speak normally and clearly. Consider that the patient might respond to you based on their own biases. Be open and honest while not assuming anything.
- Language barriers. Make sure the older adult can speak, write, and understand English. If not, obtain an interpreter other than a family member or friend.

6.15   Communication Between Caregivers and Older Adults

- Between patients and professionals
- Between patients and family members
- Between patients
- Between family members and professionals
- Between family members

As the list of communication possibilities implies, communication occurs in the health-care setting in a variety of ways.

Communication with patients occurs when a professional discusses the needs of the patient directly with the patient. This form of communication requires a two-way conversation allowing the professional as well as the patient to participate in the communication process.

Communication with family members can take place between the professional and family member; between the professional, patient, and family member; or between the patient and the family member. In all cases any discussion with the family member regarding a specific patient requires the approval of that patient. If the patient is not able to make their own decisions and has a guardian or an activated power of attorney, then the guardian or power of attorney must give permission for the professional to talk to any other family members.

Patient-Centered Communication

- The patient is at the center of the communication process.

6.16   Patient-Centered Communication

Person-centered communication focuses on the older adult as a vital member of the care team. Person-centered communication provides the opportunity for open communication and growth for both the older adult and others participating in the communication book.

- Planetree is a model of care that promotes patient-centered care which includes patient-centered communication. This philosophy promotes communication that focuses on the patient and involves the patient whenever possible. Additional information regarding Planetree can be found at http://www.planetree.org/. We will discuss Planetree in more depth later in this book.
- Eden Alternative is a philosophy of care that places the patient/resident in the center of the care team. The older adult is an integral member of the care team that builds a collaborative partnership between the older adult, the care team, and family members. Additional information regarding Eden Alternative can be found at http://www.edenalt.org/.

- Implementation of patient-centered communication requires us to listen to the older adult to find out what the older adult wants in terms of their own plan of care. The steps to implementation of person-centered communication include the following:
- Learn about the older adult including their preferences related to their own care.
- Develop a relationship of trust with the older adult by listening to what that person has to say, calling the older adult by their own name, and taking time to communicate with the older adult in a meaningful way.
- Promote the physical, psychological, and emotional well-being of the older adult by asking the individual what their needs include each time we communicate with them. For example, when the older adult puts on their call light, we need to remember they are asking for assistance and we need to approach them without judgment. Showing we care about the older adult is imperative to the communication process.
- Respect the decisions of the older adult while educating them regarding the implications of their decision. For example, if the older adult refuses to take their medication, we can educate them regarding the negative impact of this decision, but we cannot berate them or "bully" them into changing their decision. We also cannot treat the older adult like a child incapable of making decisions.

6.17   The Use of Technology in the Communication Process

6.17.1 HIPAA

- The communication process related to the older adult may include the use of technology. The use of technology requires the care providers to be diligent in terms of not only effective communication but also maintaining the older adult's privacy (HIPAA).
- Communicate with other professionals who are associated with the care of the older adult frequently to ensure each professional has adequate information to provide quality care.
- Communicate with the older adult frequently to ensure that the needs and wants of the older adult are considered and added to the overall plan of care.
- Communicate with family members (or friends) the older adult has identified. Do not communicate with family members or friends the older adult has not identified. Involve the older adult in conversations with designated family members (and/or friends) whenever possible.
- Only share the information the older adult has agreed can be shared.
- Do not leave any paperwork out for others to read. Do not walk away from a computer screen with information regarding the older adult on the screen.
- Do not use any personal devices to record, take pictures, or obtain any information regarding the older adult without the written authorization of the older adult and within facility guidelines.
- Do not discuss residents using social media

6.17.2 Technology

- *Assistive devices*: monitoring devices, hearing aids, glasses
- *PCs/laptops/social media*: Skype, Facebook, texting
- *Communication devices*: telephone amplifiers, augmentative and alternative communication such as picture boards, word boards, and voice synthesizers. Captioning devices

References

Bright Hub Education (2014) Eye contact: what does it communicate in various cultures? Retrieved from http://www.brighthubeducation.com/socialstudies-help/9626-learning-about-eye-contact-in-other-cultures/

Cotton G (2013) Gestures to avoid in cross-cultural business: in other words, "Keep your fingers to yourself". Retrieved from http://www.huffingtonpost.com/gayle-cotton/cross-cultural-gestures_b_3437653.html

Dictionary.com (2017) Homograph. Retrieved from http://www.dictionary.com/browse/homograph

Green L (2013) Stop these 7 non-verbal behaviors that are killing your career. Retrieved from https://www.pgi.com/blog/2013/03/stop-these-7-nonverbal-behaviors-that-are-killing-your-career/

Gut A, Wilczewski M, Gorbaniuk O (2017) Cultural differences, stereotypes and communication needs in intercultural communication in a global multicultural environment. J Intercult Commun 43

Institute for Healthcare Improvement (2017) SBAR: situation-background-assessment-recommendation. Publisher: Author

Lemfuss N, Prinzmetal W, Ivry R (2012) How does language change perception. A cautionary note. Front Psychol 3:78

The Joint Commission (2017) SBAR. A powerful tool to help improve communication. Retrieved from https://www.jointcommission.org/at_home_with_the_joint_commission/sbar_%e2%80%93_a_powerful_tool_to_help_improve_communication/

thebalance (2017) Nonverbal communication in the workplace. Retrieved from https://www.thebalance.com/nonverbal-communication-in-theworkplace-1918470

Thistlethwaite J (2015) Intra- and interprofessional communication. Commun Qual Saf Health Care:176–188

Vocabulary.com (2017) Homonym. Retrieved from https://www.vocabulary.com/dictionary/homonym

Suggested Reading

Mueller C, Tetzlaff B, Theile G, Fleishmann N, Cavazzini C, Geister C, Scherer M, Weyerer S, van den Bussche H, Hummers-Pradier E (2014) Interprofessional collaboration and communication in nursing homes: a qualitative exploration of problems in medical care for nursing home residents – study protocol. J Adv Nurs 71(2):451–457

Team Building and the Civil Work Environment

7

7.1 Introduction

This chapter provides information regarding the team building process and how to create a work environment that is conducive to team building. You will also learn about your role as a facilitator and collaborator. This chapter will also look at a team building process called TeamSTEPPS. Finally, the role of civility in team building will be explored as well as the detrimental impact of incivility.

7.2 Objectives

1. Identify the steps required to develop and maintain the team approach to care of the older adult.
2. Discuss the role of the LPN in the team building and maintenance process.
3. Facilitate shared decision-making model incorporating all members in a team-based model of care including staff and residents.
4. Collaborate across disciplines and shifts as well as residents and family members.
5. Identify the role of the LPN in the delegation process.
6. Identify the steps required to develop and maintain the team approach to care of the older adult.
7. Discuss the role of the LPN in the team building and maintenance process.
8. Identify issues associated with incivility.
9. Explain the role of the LPN in creating and sustaining a civil work environment.
10. Define facilitation and facilitator.
11. Explain collaboration.
12. Incivility and civility in the workplace.
13. TeamSTEPPS.

© Springer International Publishing AG 2018
C. Kruschke, *Leadership Skills for Licensed Practical Nurses Working with the Aging Population*, https://doi.org/10.1007/978-3-319-69862-5_7

7.3   The Importance of Teams in Health Care

As we have moved away from the medical model of care to the patient-centered model of care in the nursing home setting, we are finding the team approach to the provision of care is important. This is especially important as we move toward accountable care organizations, which will require partnerships between providers of care across the health-care continuum. The team approach requires organizations to understand the importance of teams and the steps necessary to the formation of teams and how to maintain the team until the team is disbanded. Leaders need to support the role of teams within the organization in order for teams to be successful (Taplin et al. 2013).

7.4   Identify the Steps Required to Develop and Maintain the Team Approach to Care of the Older Adult

The first step in the development and maintenance of a team is to define what a team is. There are a variety of team definitions that can be applied. For the purposes of this book, I will define a team as a group of individuals who come together through shared work and/or interests. This team can be decribed by the unit each person works on or a common goal, such as improving resident outcomes. Team members might include any or all of the following depending on why a team is developed and what the goals are of the team:

- Peers
- Leaders/supervisors/managers/directors
- Interdisciplinary members from different departments in the organization
- Individuals from different units
- Individuals from different shifts
- RNs, LPNs, and CNAs

The licensed practical nurse (LPN) is an important member of the care team. The LPN is often in a position of leadership in the nursing home setting, even if that position of leadership is limited to a unit. Therefore, it is important that the LPN understands how the team building concept works and what their role is in the successful development and maintenance of workplace teams.

Now that we have defined what a team is, we need to review the steps in the development of a team.

7.4.1   Selecting

The first step in the team building process is to select the individuals who need to be on the team you are forming. There are a variety of criteria you can use to determine team members. Let's look at a variety of teams based on the selection process.

- A unit team is developed based on where individuals are working in the care environment. Many organizations develop teams based on the unit where staff works. For example, if you work on a long-term care unit in your nursing home, you would develop your team based on who works in the unit, including the nurse and the certified nursing assistants. This might include all three shifts, or you could develop a separate smaller team for each shift and one primary team for the nurses and certified nursing assistants who work the unit regardless of the shift they work.
- An interdisciplinary team is developed to improve outcomes of residents/patients/clients in the health-care setting. In the nursing home, care planning team is developed as an interdisciplinary team to complete the care plan for each resident. This team also includes the resident and the resident's representative or others the resident designates as important to them.
- Person-centered care team or culture change team is developed in the health-care setting to provide direction to the organization related to meeting the requirements for pursuing culture change and person-centered care. This is an ongoing journey that is now part of requirements for the Centers for Medicare and Medicaid and The Joint Commission. Your person-centered care team should include members from the entire organization from members of leadership to members of every department. There should be a blend of managers and non-managers to ensure everyone has a voice.
- Department teams may develop to pursue objectives specific to a department. Maintenance might develop a team to implement a new program to ensure all equipment is included in an annual maintenance program. The unit care team on the third floor might be developed to pursue consistent assignments. The dietary department might develop a small work team to develop a new dish washing program.

You will find that each team is unique as described, and not everyone can or should be on each team. Base the size of the team on the objectives outlined when the team is first brought together. Most teams are developed for a specific purpose and are continued until that purpose has been fulfilled. Other teams are intended for the long term such as care planning teams. While the members of a specific care planning team may change, the care planning team itself is intended to continue as long as there are residents who need a care plan. When choosing team members, you need to consider a variety of attributes to ensure your team is as diverse as possible, which will provide the greatest opportunity for success. Consider the following attributes as you choose team members:

- Knowledge, skills, and abilities or attitudes
- Background
- Stakeholders
- Work styles
- Diversity of roles, backgrounds, and traits (Ulrich and Manning Crider 2017)
- Multigenerational (Moore et al. 2016)

Now we need to look at how teams are formed.

7.4.2   Forming

The team is formed as soon as a group of individuals begin working together. There needs to be someone designated as the leader for the group. This person is important to the group for the following reasons:

- Make sure the group follows the objectives of the team.
- Keep group discussions on task rather than digressing to other topics.
- Ensure the group meets as often as needed to meet the team objectives.

When the team first comes together, members may not know each other very well. The first meeting of the team would be an appropriate opportunity for each member to introduce themselves to the other team members. The leader can decide how much information is necessary for the other members to know. The leader also needs to share the common goals of the team or start the team relationship by having the team members develop the shared goals of the team. The shared goals of the team must be developed prior to any other decisions being made. The next step is to determine the outcomes of the team based on the goals of the team and the timeline for completion (Ulrich and Manning Crider 2017). Your role as an LPN leader provides the opportunity for you to share the goals of the team as it is formed.

7.4.3   Storming

From the very beginning of the team, you will find that the team does not always work in unison. The term *storming* is used as a term to describe the "growing pains" of the team. I call this "growing pains" because team development requires a group of individuals to work together toward a common goal or goals who may or may not know each other (Ulrich and Manning Crider, 2017). When we have to develop relationships at work that are not necessarily relationships we would have chosen on our own, we will find that there can be storm clouds as each individual on the team expresses themselves independently of other team members. This may also occur when decisions are made and one or more members of the team do not agree, resulting in pushback as the decisions are implemented. This does not make the team member or members bad individuals. Sometimes this is how individuals react when they do not feel they are being heard. When decisions are made they do not agree with, this may lead to feelings of not being heard. It will take time to work through these issues and help the individual or individuals understand that there does not always need to be agreement to work together. Team members need support to understand their role and it is acceptable to disagree, with the important understanding the common goals of the team must take priority over individual goals.

Other aspects needing to be taken into consideration include team members who do not like other team members, differing personalities and work styles that may precipitate conflict, or one or more members who challenge the authority of the team leader. In these cases the team leader may need to work with individual team members to help them gain perspective on the role of the team as compared to the role of the team member. Team members need to be reassured they do not need to like someone else on the team to work with the team. But, they do need to be aware of how they feel to ensure decisions they make are beneficial to the team and are not based on how they feel about a certain team member. The team leader has a responsibility to work with the team and develop an understanding of each team member's personality and work with the strengths of each team member and their work styles. For example, if someone is a hard worker but has a difficult time with deadlines, the leader might assign tasks to that individual but assign someone else responsibility for keeping deadlines. If someone else does not like multitasking but is great at developing timelines, this would be the person to put in charge of keeping the team on-task to meet deadlines but is only given this responsibility. Remember, as a leader, you have the responsibility to make sure each team member has a voice so that one person does not take control of the team to fulfill personal agendas.

7.4.4   Norming

Norming occurs when the team comes together and works more cohesively especially related to the goals of the team. Team members have gotten to know each other and found their own place within the team. Differences of opinion are less important, and the overall goals of the team are now the priority for the team members (Ulrich and Manning Crider, 2017). There is more respect from one team member to another even in cases where team members may not have liked each other initially. While team members who have not gotten along may not become friends, there is a respectful connection for the goals of the team. The team members have come to respect the leader especially related to the work within the team and moving toward the team's goals. Team members have also developed a better understanding of more constructive ways to provide feedback that does not begin with the pronoun "you." Rather, the team member might approach a disagreement by stating, "please help me understand your position" rather than saying "you are wrong." This is an opportunity for you to show your leadership skills by exhibiting the cohesiveness you expect others to exhibit.

7.4.5   Performing

As the team moves into the *performing stage*, the team's goals are being achieved. The team has developed a cohesiveness that transcends the number of members in the team. The team needs to function longer as all of the goals are achieved (Ulrich and Manning Crider, 2017). When the team has achieved all of the goals, the team needs to determine if it is still necessary for the team to exist. If the team needs to continue to exist due to additional goals that have been developed, the team will continue. If the team no longer needs to exist because all goals have been met and no new goals have been developed, the team moves into the adjourning phase. At this point of the team's existence, you need to help the team members determine if the team is necessary beyond the completion of the original goals.

7.4.6 Adjourning

In the adjourning phase, the team is disbanded if all the goals have been met, and the team is no longer needed. Adjournment may also take place temporarily if the team will need to continue but is not needed currently. This type of adjournment is for a specific period of time rather than permanently. This is a difficult phase of the team for those who have developed relationships as part of the team, while others may feel a sense of relief that this "job" is done. Regardless, the leader of the team does need to take time to acknowledge the efforts of the team and thank them for their time and energy to complete the goals of the team (Ulrich and Manning Crider, 2017).

7.5 Team Facilitator

The team facilitator is usually the team leader as described previously but can also be a separate role to support the team to complete the goals of the team (Aga, Nooderhaven and Vallejo, 2016). When a facilitator is part of the team, the facilitator does not complete the activities of the team. Consider the following activities the team facilitator will oversee as part of the facilitator role:

- Ensure all meetings of the team are scheduled appropriately in a location that is conducive to completing the goals of the team.
- Maintain communication between team members (Brown et al, 2005).
- Facilitate team meetings by reviewing the agenda and goals of the team along with current accomplishments.
- Keep the team engaged and on track.
- Build relationships with team members (Brown et al, 2005).

The licensed practical nurse (LPN) has the ability to be a team facilitator due to the management experience obtained as a unit nurse.

7.6 Team Collaboration

Successful teams develop and maintain an environment conducive to collaboration especially interdisciplinary collaboration (Boughzala and De Vreede 2015). Team collaboration occurs when the team members work together to meet goals and expectations. With team building steps, collaboration is at its peak during the norming and performing stages. Collaboration can also occur when there are interdisciplinary members on the team such as a care planning team or the team invites input from members of the interdisciplinary team even if there are no members from a specific discipline on the team. This is especially valuable in situations where the team is working on goals and needs input from an expert in a field other than those represented by the team members. If this is the case, individuals who have the expertise needed would be invited to join the team. This addition can be for a limited period of time or permanent based on the needs of the team.

The licensed practical nurse (LPN) has the knowledge, skills, and attitude to assist the team with collaboration based on the experience of the LPN with team membership. This is especially noted with the care planning team. The LPN has knowledge of the disciplines within the nursing home setting and who to contact if additional team members are needed or the team needs specific information.

One of the most important teams in the nursing home is the care plan team. For many LPNs this is the team you will most likely be part of especially the care plan teams associated with the residents living on your unit. The care planning team must be interdisciplinary and not just the nurse, social worker, and dietician. You need to include members of the interdisciplinary team with knowledge regarding the residents and who can provide the necessary input to develop a living care plan document for each resident. Members would include the following disciplines:

- Nursing
- Social Services
- Dietary/nutrition
- Therapy
- Activities

Additional members include the unit supervisor, the certified nursing assistants who are members of the care team for the resident, the resident, and the resident's representative. You may also include housekeeping, maintenance, and laundry as needed. Care planning teams evolve from one care planning meeting to the next, shifting membership as needed. If the LPN is the nurse on the unit, the LPN will bring the care planning team together as required. However, the LPN does not have to run each care planning meeting. This role can be shifted from one member to another each time the team meets to give everyone the opportunity to lead the team. This would include the resident and/or family members.

Additional teams the LPN should consider becoming part of includes wound teams, fall prevention teams and quality improvement teams. Participation in specific teams provides the LPN with growth potential especially when the team is interdisciplinary in nature.

7.7 Dysfunctional Teams

Understanding dysfunctional teams is important in order to fully understand how to support teams to function well (Havig et al, 2013). According to Ulrich and Manning Crider (2017), there are five elements that make for a dysfunctional team.

7.7.1   Lack of Trust

If one or more members of the team do not trust other members of the team, the level of distrust climbs resulting in the team members not feeling comfortable to work within the confines of the team. This will result in lack of cohesion, and the team is not able to reach the norming and performing stages of the team. Lack of trust can result in team members leaving the team. When team members leave, the team is disrupted making it difficult for the team to reach its goals.

7.7.2   Fear of Commitment

Fear of commitment results in having team members who are so concerned regarding the dynamics of the team that they are not willing to commit to the team. This results in the team having difficulty reaching the norming and performing stages. Another aspect of fear of commitment is when one or more team members do not agree with the goals of the team but feel they do not have a voice and remain silent. Fear of commitment continues to grow unless the leader or facilitator is able to pick up on the fear of commitment and is able to support team members to overcome their fear and begin to commit to the team.

7.7.3   Avoiding Accountability

Accountability by team members and the team as a whole is very important to the success of the team. The team leader or facilitator needs to set the stage in the forming stage of the team to ensure there is commitment to the goals of the team and accountability regarding which team member(s) will be responsible for which aspects of the team's goals. If there is no accountability, there is the possibility the team will be less successful in fulfillment of the team goals.

7.7.4   Lack of Attention to Result

Lack of attention to results can result in the team not meeting the required goals of the team or missing elements of the goals. For example, if team members are not attentive to the team results, one or more elements of the results could be missed resulting in the team being less successful. An example would be if team members are not focused on due dates and miss a due date for one or more of the team's goals.

7.7.5   Groupthink

Groupthink must be considered when reviewing dysfunctional teams. Groupthink occurs when team members acquiesce to decisions based on what they believe the team wants rather than giving an alternative opinion. For example, if the team wants to finish a project which requires a vote, members of the team may vote in favor of the project even if they do not agree in order for the project to be accepted and the team to meet its objectives. As pointed out by Ulrich and Manning Crider (2017), groupthink gives the allusion of cohesiveness even though cohesiveness does not exist. One step the leader or facilitator can take to avoid groupthink is to make sure each member of the team is verbal regarding their own opinions with an emphasis on stating why they feel the way they do. The LPN as facilitator should share their own opinions with the team to emulate the behavior they are looking for in the other team members.

7.8   TeamSTEPPS

The Agency for Healthcare Research and Quality (AHRQ) (2017) has teamed up with the Department of Defense to develop TeamSTEPPS. This initiative is intended to assist organizations in the development of the team approach. According to AHRQ (2017), the development of the team approach to the provision of care results in a safe environment for the residents and staff. The premise of TeamSTEPPS can be applied to the development of teams regardless of the objectives of the team. TeamSTEPPS is evidence based and can be applied to any health-care setting in the development of teams. There is a specific TeamSTEPPS curriculum for long-term care, and this curriculum can be found at https://www.ahrq.gov/teamstepps/longtermcare/index.html. There are 11 modules in the curriculum as well as a supplemental module. Review the curriculum to determine if this program would be of interest to you and/or members of your leadership team within your organization.

7.9   Civility in the Workplace

Team building requires an environment that is conducive to the growth of employees and team building. When the work environment is less than civil, the ability to work together can be compromised.

7.9.1   Incivility

Incivility in the workplace is a lack of respect for fellow workers that manifests itself in a variety of ways. Behaviors that can be considered uncivil include the following:

- Making derogatory comments
- Rolling the eyes when someone else is speaking
- Criticism in public
- Making comments of a personal nature that are considered rude or derogatory
- Raising your voice

- Making off-color jokes at the expense of someone based on their ethnicity, gender, religion, age, etc.
- Negative behavior that is sustained (Lachman 2014)

The American Nurses Association's Code of Ethics for Nurses indicates incivility is unethical behavior (Lachman 2014). We need to all work together to avoid incivility. We need to remember incivility is not appropriate and can lead to job dissatisfaction, low morale, and ultimately an increase in turnover. According to Lachman (2014), The Joint Commission issued a statement that incivility could lead to a decline in safety, including patient and staff safety. With continued incivility, patient satisfaction and patient outcomes will decline. With the decline in staff satisfaction and patient satisfaction, the organization will be impacted financially when reimbursement is reduced due to the decline in overall satisfaction.

The American Nurses Association (2015) has updated their position regarding incivility in the workplace. The overarching theme of this position paper is that the nursing profession as a whole would not tolerate violence of any kind by anyone. The American Nurses Association provides a variety of resources related to workplace violence at http://www.nursingworld.org/Bullying-Workplace-Violence.

The Centers for Disease Control and Prevention (2016) has developed education titled "Workplace Violence Prevention for Nurses," which can be accessed at https://wwwn.cdc.gov/wpvhc/Course.aspx/Slide/Intro_1. This education provides information regarding workplace violence, prevention strategies, and intervention strategies.

The important understanding regarding incivility and workplace violence is that this type of behavior is not acceptable or ethical. As a LPN, you have a responsibility to learn as much as you can about incivility and workplace violence and advocate for education of all staff regarding these issues. With education, a civil workplace environment is achievable.

References

Aga D, Noorderhaven N, Vallejo B (2016) Transformational leadership and project success: The mediating role of team building. International Journal of Project Management, 34:806–818

Agency for Healthcare Research and Quality (2017) TeamSTEPPS long term care version. Retrieved from https://www.ahrq.gov/teamstepps/longtermcare/index.html

American Nurses Association (2015) Incivility, bullying, and workplace violence. Retrieved from http://www.nursingworld.org/Bullying-Workplace-Violence

Boughzala I, De Vreede G (2015) Evaluating team coillaboration quality: the development and field application of a collaboration maturity model. J Manag Info Syst 32(3):129–157

Brown C, Holcomb L, Maloney J, Naranjo J, Gibson C, Russell P (2005) Caring in action: the patient care facilitator role. Int J Hum Car 9(3):51–58

Centers for Disease Control and Prevention (2016) Workplace violence prevention for nurses. Retrieved from https://wwwn.cdc.gov/wpvhc/Course.aspx/Slide/Intro_1

Havig A, Skogstad A, Veensta M, Romoren T (2013) Real teams and their effect on the quality of care in nursing homes. BMC Health Serv Res 13:499. https://doi.org/10.1186/1472-6963-13-499.

Lachman V (2014) Ethical issues in the disruptive behaviors of incivility, bullying, and horizontal/lateral violence. Medsurg Nurs 23(1):56–60

Moore J, Everly M, Bauer R (2016) Multigenerational challenges: team-building for positive clinical workforce outcomes. Online J Issues Nurs 21(2):3

Taplin S, Foster M, Shortell S (2013) Organizational leadership for building effective health care teams. Ann Fam Med 11(3):279–281

Ulrich B, Manning Crider N (2017) Using teams to improve outcomes and performance. Nephrol Nurs J 44(2):141–151

Quality Improvement

8

8.1 Introduction

The role of the Licensed Practical Nurse (LPN) continues to expand in the long term care setting. Part of this expansion, is the growth of quality improvement to meet regulatory compliance. With LPNs leading in the care of the aging population within the long term care setting, it is no surprise that LPNs need to understand quality improvement and their leadership role to ensure quality and safety. Understanding quality improvement and safety begins with understanding the role of QSEN in this process.

8.2 Objectives

1. Discuss quality improvement and identify areas that need improvement.
2. Explain the role of QSEN in maintaining quality and safety.

8.3 Quality and Safety Education for Nurses (QSEN)

Following the release of the seminal work, *To Error is Human: Building a Safer Health System*, the Quality and Safety Education for Nurses (QSEN) was implemented to improve quality in health care. This initiative was intended to educate nurses regarding the competencies associated with quality and safety within the health care environment (AORN, 2017). According to Dolansky and Moore (2013), nurses need to move beyond the application of QSEN on an individual level to a more comprehensive system-thinking approach that takes into consideration how each decision not only impacts one person, but how these decisions will impact the system (Way and McKeeby, 2008). We can consider this at the nursing home level by considering how our decisions as nurses not only impact each resident on our

© Springer International Publishing AG 2018   95
C. Kruschke, *Leadership Skills for Licensed Practical Nurses Working with the Aging Population*, https://doi.org/10.1007/978-3-319-69862-5_8

unit but all the residents in the nursing home. Developing quality improvement and safety initiatives must expand to incorporate the entire system.

Quality and safety education includes the following:

- Patient-centered care
- Team work and collaboration
- Evidence-based practice
- Quality improvement
- Safety
- Informatics (Webster University, 2017)

When considering patient-centered care you need to consider that your residents have a right to participate in all decision-making for their own care. Team work and collaboration are an important part of the decision-making process as interdisciplinary members come together to achieve quality care for all residents. When we consider quality care we need to review current practice as compared to research that outlines best practices. This information needs to be combined with the rights of the residents and/or their resident designee to ensure the residents have a voice in their own care (Ironside, 2007). As you are learning in this chapter, continuous quality improvement is required to ensure you are meeting all the regulatory and legal requirements for resident care that encompasses current standards. This includes the safety concerns associated with quality resident care as well as the safety of the care providers. This includes the use of informatics as a means to communicate rationales for decision-making (QSEN Institute 2017; Hunt, 2012). Table 8.1 QSEN Competencies has been reproduced from Cronenwett et al. (2007) with permission from Elsevier, LTD. This table combines six separate tables from the original article, Quality and Safety Education for Nurses into Table 8.1 QSEN Competencies. To use this table, review each category including the following:

- Category title
- Definition
- Knowledge
- Skills
- Attitudes

Compare the information provided in the table for each category to your current knowledge, skills and attitudes. If you find there is a gap in your own knowledge, skills and attitudes; refer your concerns to the Staff Development Coordinator or the individual assigned to staff development. Having a better understanding of these categories prepares you for systems thinking.

Table 8.1   QSEN competencies

Knowledge	Skills	Attitudes
Table 1: Patient-centered care		
Definition: Recognize the patient or designee as the source of control and full partner in providing compassionate and coordinated care based on respect for patient's preferences, values, and needs		
Integrate understanding of multiple dimensions of patient centered care: • Patient/family/community preferences, values • Coordination and integration of care • Information, communication, and education • Physical comfort and emotional support • Involvement of family and friends • Transition and continuity Describe how diverse cultural, ethnic and social backgrounds function as sources of patient, family, and community values	Elicit patient values, preferences and expressed needs as part of clinical interview, implementation of care plan and evaluation of care Communicate patient values, preferences and expressed needs to other members of health care team Provide patient-centered care with sensitivity and respect for the diversity of human experience	Value seeing health care situations "through patients' eyes" Respect and encourage individual expression of patient values, preferences and expressed needs Value the patient's expertise with own health and symptoms Seek learning opportunities with patients who represent all aspects of human diversity Recognize personally held attitudes about working with patients from different ethnic, cultural and social backgrounds Willingly support patient-centered care for individuals and groups whose values differ from own
Demonstrate comprehensive understanding of the concepts of pain and suffering, including physiologic models of pain and comfort	Assess presence and extent of pain and suffering Assess levels of physical and emotional comfort Elicit expectations of patient & family for relief of pain, discomfort, or suffering Initiate effective treatments to relieve pain and suffering in light of patient values, preferences and expressed needs	Recognize personally held values and beliefs about the management of pain or suffering Appreciate the role of the nurse in relief of all types and sources of pain or suffering Recognize that patient expectations influence outcomes in management of pain or suffering
Examine how the safety, quality and cost effectiveness of health care can be improved through the active involvement of patients and families Examine common barriers to active involvement of patients in their own health care processes Describe strategies to empower patients or families in all aspects of the health care process	Remove barriers to presence of families and other designated surrogates based on patient preferences Assess level of patient's decisional conflict and provide access to resources Engage patients or designated surrogates in active partnerships that promote health, safety and well-being, and self-care management	Value active partnership with patients or designated surrogates in planning, implementation, and evaluation of care Respect patient preferences for degree of active engagement in care process Respect patient's right to access to personal health records

(continued)

Table 8.1   (continued)

Knowledge	Skills	Attitudes
Explore ethical and legal implications of patient-centered care Describe the limits and boundaries of therapeutic patient-centered care	Recognize the boundaries of therapeutic relationships Facilitate informed patient consent for care	Acknowledge the tension that may exist between patient rights and the organizational responsibility for professional, ethical care Appreciate shared decision-making with empowered patients and families, even when conflicts occur
Discuss principles of effective communication Describe basic principles of consensus building and conflict resolution Examine nursing roles in assuring coordination, integration, and continuity of care	Assess own level of communication skill in encounters with patients and families Participate in building consensus or resolving conflict in the context of patient care Communicate care provided and needed at each transition in care	Value continuous improvement of own communication and conflict resolution skills

Table 2: Teamwork and collaboration

Definition: Function effectively within nursing and inter-professional teams, fostering open communication, mutual respect, and shared decision-making to achieve quality patient care		
Describe own strengths, limitations, and values in functioning as a member of a team	Demonstrate awareness of own strengths and limitations as a team member Initiate plan for self-development as a team member Act with integrity, consistency and respect for differing views	Acknowledge own potential to contribute to effective team functioning Appreciate importance of intra- and inter-professional collaboration
Describe scopes of practice and roles of health care team members Describe strategies for identifying and managing overlaps in team member roles and accountabilities Recognize contributions of other individuals and groups in helping patient/family achieve health goals	Function competently within own scope of practice as a member of the health care team Assume role of team member or leader based on the situation Initiate requests for help when appropriate to situation Clarify roles and accountabilities under conditions of potential overlap in team member functioning Integrate the contributions of others who play a role in helping patient/family achieve health goals	Value the perspectives and expertise of all health team members Respect the centrality of the patient/family as core members of any health care team Respect the unique attributes that members bring to a team, including variations in professional orientations and accountabilities

Table 8.1 (continued)

Knowledge	Skills	Attitudes
Analyze differences in communication style preferences among patients and families, nurses and other members of the health team Describe impact of own communication style on others Discuss effective strategies for communicating and resolving conflict	Communicate with team members, adapting own style of communicating to needs of the team and situation Demonstrate commitment to team goals Solicit input from other team members to improve individual, as well as team, performance Initiate actions to resolve conflict	Value teamwork and the relationships upon which it is based Value different styles of communication used by patients, families and health care providers Contribute to resolution of conflict and disagreement
Describe examples of the impact of team functioning on safety and quality of care Explain how authority gradients influence teamwork and patient safety	Follow communication practices that minimize risks associated with handoffs among providers and across transitions in care Assert own position/perspective in discussions about patient care Choose communication styles that diminish the risks associated with authority gradients among team members	Appreciate the risks associated with handoffs among providers and across transitions in care
Identify system barriers and facilitators of effective team functioning Examine strategies for improving systems to support team functioning	Participate in designing systems that support effective teamwork	Value the influence of system solutions in achieving effective team functioning
Table 3: Evidence-based practice (EBP)		
Definition: Integrate best current evidence with clinical expertise and patient/family preferences and values for delivery of optimal health care		
Demonstrate knowledge of basic scientific methods and processes Describe EBP to include the components of research evidence, clinical expertise and patient/family values	Participate effectively in appropriate data collection and other research activities Adhere to institutional review board (IRB) guidelines Base individualized care plan on patient values, clinical expertise and evidence	Appreciate strengths and weaknesses of scientific bases for practice Value the need for ethical conduct of research and quality improvement Value the concept of EBP as integral to determining best clinical practice

(continued)

Table 8.1 (continued)

Knowledge	Skills	Attitudes
Differentiate clinical opinion from research and evidence summaries Describe reliable sources for locating evidence reports and clinical practice guidelines	Read original research and evidence reports related to area of practice Locate evidence reports related to clinical practice topics and guidelines	Appreciate the importance of regularly reading relevant professional journals
Explain the role of evidence in determining best clinical practice Describe how the strength and relevance of available evidence influences the choice of interventions in provision of patient-centered care	Participate in structuring the work environment to facilitate integration of new evidence into standards of practice Question rationale for routine approaches to care that result in less-than-desired outcomes or adverse events	Value the need for continuous improvement in clinical practice based on new knowledge
Discriminate between valid and invalid reasons for modifying evidence-based clinical practice based on clinical expertise or patient/family preferences	Consult with clinical experts before deciding to deviate from evidence-based protocols	Acknowledge own limitations in knowledge and clinical expertise before determining when to deviate from evidence-based best practices

Table 4: Quality improvement (QI)

Definition: Use data to monitor the outcomes of care processes and use improvement methods to design and test changes to continuously improve the quality and safety of health care systems

Knowledge	Skills	Attitudes
Describe strategies for learning about the outcomes of care in the setting in which one is engaged in clinical practice	Seek information about outcomes of care for populations served in care setting Seek information about quality improvement projects in the care setting	Appreciate that continuous quality improvement is an essential part of the daily work of all health professionals
Recognize that nursing and other health professions students are parts of systems of care and care processes that affect outcomes for patients and families Give examples of the tension between professional autonomy and system functioning	Use tools (such as flow charts, cause-effect diagrams) to make processes of care explicit Participate in a root cause analysis of a sentinel event	Value own and others' contributions to outcomes of care in local care settings
Explain the importance of variation and measurement in assessing quality of care	Use quality measures to understand performance Use tools (such as control charts and run charts) that are helpful for understanding variation Identify gaps between local and best practice	Appreciate how unwanted variation affects care Value measurement and its role in good patient care

Table 8.1 (continued)

Knowledge	Skills	Attitudes
Describe approaches for changing processes of care	Design a small test of change in daily work (using an experiential learning method such as Plan-Do-Study-Act) Practice aligning the aims, measures and changes involved in improving care Use measures to evaluate the effect of change	Value local change (in individual practice or team practice on a unit) and its role in creating joy in work Appreciate the value of what individuals and teams can to do to improve care

Table 5: Safety

Definition: Minimizes risk of harm to patients and providers through both system effectiveness and individual performance

Knowledge	Skills	Attitudes
Examine human factors and other basic safety design principles as well as commonly used unsafe practices (such as, work-arounds and dangerous abbreviations) Describe the benefits and limitations of selected safety-enhancing technologies (such as, barcodes, Computer Provider Order Entry, medication pumps, and automatic alerts/alarms) Discuss effective strategies to reduce reliance on memory	Demonstrate effective use of technology and standardized practices that support safety and quality Demonstrate effective use of strategies to reduce risk of harm to self or others Use appropriate strategies to reduce reliance on memory (such as, forcing functions, checklists)	Value the contributions of standardization/reliability to safety Appreciate the cognitive and physical limits of human performance
Delineate general categories of errors and hazards in care Describe factors that create a culture of safety (such as, open communication strategies and organizational error reporting systems)	Communicate observations or concerns related to hazards and errors to patients, families and the health care team Use organizational error reporting systems for near miss and error reporting	Value own role in preventing errors
Describe processes used in understanding causes of error and allocation of responsibility and accountability (such as, root cause analysis and failure mode effects analysis)	Participate appropriately in analyzing errors and designing system improvements Engage in root cause analysis rather than blaming when errors or near misses occur	Value vigilance and monitoring (even of own performance of care activities) by patients, families, and other members of the health care team
Discuss potential and actual impact of national patient safety resources, initiatives and regulations	Use national patient safety resources for own professional development and to focus attention on safety in care settings	Value relationship between national safety campaigns and implementation in local practices and practice settings

(continued)

Table 8.1   (continued)

Knowledge	Skills	Attitudes
Table 6: Informatics		
Definition: Use information and technology to communicate, manage knowledge, mitigate error, and support decision making		
Explain why information and technology skills are essential for safe patient care	Seek education about how information is managed in care settings before providing care Apply technology and information management tools to support safe processes of care	Appreciate the necessity for all health professionals to seek lifelong, continuous learning of information technology skills
Identify essential information that must be available in a common database to support patient care Contrast benefits and limitations of different communication technologies and their impact on safety and quality	Navigate the electronic health record Document and plan patient care in an electronic health record Employ communication technologies to coordinate care for patients	Value technologies that support clinical decision-making, error prevention, and care coordination Protect confidentiality of protected health information in electronic health records
Describe examples of how technology and information management are related to the quality and safety of patient care Recognize the time, effort, and skill required for computers, databases and other technologies to become reliable and effective tools for patient care	Respond appropriately to clinical decision-making supports and alerts Use information management tools to monitor outcomes of care processes Use high quality electronic sources of healthcare information	Value nurses' involvement in design, selection, implementation, and evaluation of information technologies to support patient care

Cronenwett, L., Sherwood, G., Barnsteiner, J., Disch, J., Johnson, J., Mitchell, P., Taylor Sullivan, D., and Warren, J. (2007). Quality and safety education for nurses. *Nursing Outlook*; 55: 122-131.

8.4   Systems Thinking

Systems thinking involves the ability of leaders and managers to see the links between one element of the system to all other aspects of the system. (The Institute for Systematic Leadership 2017). Consider the nursing home environment as a complete system. You are the manager on one unit in the nursing home system. Your unit would be considered one element of the system. Another unit would be considered another element of the system. Each department within the nursing home (e.g., dietary, social services, maintenance, etc.) are each considered one element of the nursing home system. When you use systems thinking, you are considering how decisions you make on your unit impact other areas of the nursing home.

Consider the following examples of decisions that might impact other units or departments within your nursing home:

1. You decide to have breakfast served on your unit 30 min later every morning.
2. You make the decision to use consistent assignments on your unit even though all other units do not use consistent assignments.
3. You make the decision to have your certified nursing assistants develop their own schedules.

When you consider each of these decisions, you may or may not see the connection to other units. We need to consider each of these decisions separately to make those important connections.

You decide to have breakfast served on your unit 30 min later every morning

While this decision may appear to impact only your unit, consider the following:

- If your unit is being served breakfast 30 min later every day, other units are impacted because their breakfast schedule may be altered in order to allow your unit to be served later. The unit served 30 min after your unit will now have to be served earlier than your unit or even later than previously served to allow your unit to move into their time slot.
- Dietary will need to change their schedule to ensure your unit receives breakfast 30 min later. This might mean another unit must be served earlier or all units will be saved later. If all units are served later, dietary staff schedules will need to be changed to make sure staff are available to stay later. To avoid overtime, this will mean the staff will have to come in later. This could impact other units that are served before your unit. You can now see the impact of this decision on one department.
- Housekeeping staff will need to be made aware of this change so that housekeeping avoids cleaning on your unit while breakfast is being served. This will impact their overall cleaning schedule in order to make the necessary adjustments.
- Maintenance staff will need to be made aware of this change so that the maintenance staff avoids making repairs on your unit while breakfast is being served. This has the potential to alter their schedule if repairs on your unit need to be done earlier or later than the current schedule.
- Therapy staff need to be aware of this change so that therapy sessions are not scheduled during breakfast. In addition, if therapy staff are walking residents to the dining room for meals as part of their therapy program, the change in the breakfast schedule will impact the schedule of therapists who provide therapy during the time breakfast will now be served on your unit.
- How will this decision impact other units or departments in your nursing home?

You make the decision to use consistent assignments on your unit even though all other units do not use consistent assignments

You may or may not consider a decision you make on your unit regarding consistent assistant assignments as an issue that would impact other units. Consider the following questions:

- If the certified nursing assistants on your unit have consistent assignments and other units do not, how will this impact other certified nursing assistants who would like consistent assignments?
- How will other nurses feel if they are forced to switch to consistent assignments?
- If you make this decision without input from leadership, will your decision be reversed by a leader if they are not in agreement?

You make the decision to have your certified nursing assistants develop their own schedules

The same questions and concerns can be applied to this decision. In addition, consider the following questions:

- How will the change in scheduling impact weekends and holidays?
- How will the change in scheduling impact overtime?
- Will you have enough staff to cover all openings on your schedule?
- What if there is no certified nursing assistant who wants to work specific shifts of days of the week?
- How will you cover holes in your schedule?

When considering decisions you are going to make related to quality improvement, you need to take systems thinking into consideration. Any decision made in one area of the nursing home should be considered for feasibility in any or all other areas of the nursing home.

8.5   Quality Improvement and Identify Areas that Need Improvement

1. Developing a safe environment
   (a) Resident safety refers to development of a program to ensure the safety of the residents. This includes safety from incidents and accidents. The Centers for Medicare and Medicaid Services issued a final ruling regarding improvements in safety for nursing home residents. The goals of this final rule are to reduce hospital re-admissions, reduce infections, and improve quality of care received by the residents and increased safety measures in the nursing home setting. The final rulings related to resident safety include the following:
   - Staff are properly trained to prevent elder abuse.
   - When staffing the nursing home, the health of the residents need to be taken into consideration to ensure there are enough staff to properly care for the residents.

- Staff have the appropriate training and skills necessary to provide person-centered care.
- Discharge planning to include education of residents regarding their needs following discharge and appropriate discharge information is provided to the facility the resident is discharged to or the service provider the resident will need following discharge.
- Nursing homes are required to update their infection prevention and control program to include the requirement that the nursing home have an infection prevention and control officer as well as an antibiotic stewardship program (Centers for Medicare and Medicaid Services 2016).

The Joint Commission has developed national patient safety goals for nursing homes including the following:

- Identify residents correctly.
- Safe Medication Management related to anticoagulant therapy.
- Infection prevention.
- Prevent residents from falling.
- Prevention of bed sores (The Joint Commission 2017).
    - (b) Staff safety refers to development of a program to ensure the safety of the staff especially those who provide direct resident care.
    - (c) Risk Management in the long term care setting refers to understanding the risks.
    - (d) Restraint-free environment refers to the ruling in the 1987 Nursing Home Reform Act passed by Congress requiring nursing homes to refrain from using unnecessary chemical or physical restraints on residents. This began the quality improvement initiative to reduce and eliminate chemical and physical restraints unless medically necessary. In most cases, this initiative resulted in restraint reduction. Alternative approaches to the use of restraints were initiated with excellent results. Now, alternative approaches are initiated rather than using restraints. If restraints need to be used, a restraint reduction program must also be initiated in order to reduce and eliminate the restraint as soon as possible. If the restraint is not able to be reduced or eliminated, the restraint must be care planned and documentation must reflect the efforts tried. To ensure this process continues any use of restraints must be reported to CMS as part of the completion of the Minimum Data Set (MDS). When a nursing home is using any type of restraint, the use must be investigated through the survey process and reviewed for relevance. We have seen a reduction in use of restraints from 21.1% in 1991 to 5% in 2007 (Center for Medicare and Medicaid Services 2008, p. 8).
    - (e) Falls reduction. As discussed previously, falls reduction is part of safety programs in the nursing home setting.
2. Adverse Events in Nursing Homes. The Centers for Medicare and Medicaid Services has developed programming to assist nursing homes to identify, track and investigate adverse events that have already occurred as well as development of program interventions to prevent adverse events. The Office of Inspector General has identified that 60% of adverse events in nursing homes were

preventable. The Office of Inspector General went on to report that 37% of adverse events were related to medication management. The Centers for Medicare and Medicaid services worked with the Agency for healthcare Research and Quality to develop an Adverse Drug Event Trigger Tool intended to look at preventable adverse drug events, risk factors associated with preventable adverse drug events, triggers and systems for surveyors to evaluate adverse drug event prevention programs.

The Centers for Disease Control and Prevention (CDC) developed an Infection Control Assessment Tool for Long-Term Care Facilities based on the research indicating that at least 30% of adverse events were related to development of infections in the long term care setting. This tool is intended to assist nursing homes in the evaluation of their infection control program. https://www.cms.gov/Medicare/Provider-Enrollment-and-Certification/QAPI/Adverse-Events-NHs.html.
(a) Definition
(b) Impact on long term care

8.6   QAPI and Quality Improvement

Nursing Home Survey on Patient Safety Culture, https://www.ahrq.gov/professionals/quality-patient-safety/patientsafetyculture/nursing-home/index.html   provides additional information regarding nursing home culture of patient safety.

References

AORN (2017). Quality and Safety Education for Nurses (QSEN). Retrieved from https://www.aorn.org/education/facility-solutions/periop-101/qsen
Centers for Medicare and Medicaid (2008) Freedom from unnecessary physical restraints: two decades of national progress in nursing home care. Publisher: Author. Retrieved from https://www.cms.gov/site-search/search-results.html?q=restraint%20free
Centers for Medicare and Medicaid (2016). CMS finalizes improvements in care, safety, and consumer protections for long-term care facility residents. Retrieved from https://www.cms.gov/Newsroom/MediaReleaseDatabase/Press-releases/2016-Press-releases-items/2016-09-28.html
Cronenwett L, Sherwood G, Barnsteiner J, Disch J, Johnson J, Mitchell P, Taylor Sullivan D, and Warren J (2007) Quality and safety education for nurses. Nursing Outlook 55:122–131
Dolansky M, Moore S (2013) Quality and safety education for nurses (QSEN): the key is systems thinking. The ANA periodicals. Online J Issues Nurs 18(3):1
Health Information Technology (HITS) (n.d.) for nursing faculty: QSEN: quality and safety competencies. http://libguides.webster.edu/c.php?g=98020&p=633889
Hunt D (2012) QSEN competencies: A bridge to practice. Nursing Made Incredibly Easy! 10(5):1–3. doi:10.1097/01.NME.0000418040.92006.70. Retrieved from http://journals.lww.com/nursingmadeincrediblyeasy/Fulltext/2012/09000/QSEN_competencies__A_bridge_to_practice.1.aspx
Ironside, P (2007). Exploring the complexity of advocacy: balancing patient-centered care and safety. Retrieved from http://www.qsen.org/teachingstrategy.php?id=58

QSEN Institute (2017) QSEN competencies. Retrieved from http://qsen.org/competencies/pre-licensure-ksas/

The Joint Commission (2017). Nursing care center national patient safety goals. Retrieved from https://www.jointcommission.org/ncc_2017_npsgs/

The Institute for Systems Thinking (2017). Basic principles of systems thinking as applied to management and leadership. Retrieved from http://www.systemicleadershipinstitute.org/systemic-leadership/theories/basic-principles-of-systems-thinking-as-applied-to-management-andleadership-2/

Way C, and McKeeby J (2008) Systems thinking as a team-building approach. The Systems Thinker, 19(8):44–49

Webster University (2017). Health Information Technology (HITS) for Nursing Faculty: QSEN: Quality and Safety Competencies. Retrieved from http://libguides.webster.edu/c.php?g=98020&p=633889

Aspects Integral to Managing the Care Environment

9

9.1 Introduction

This chapter provides you with the opportunity to learn more about the management process in relationship to the care environment where our aging population lives. This chapter also reviews your role in the management process.

9.2 Objectives

- Identify the role of the LPN in a variety of settings:
  - Acute care
  - Nursing home
  - Assisted living
  - Home health
- Identify the role of the LPN in the delegation process

9.3 The Role of the LPN in the Acute Care Setting

Depending on the education you received and the state you live in will dictate the role you take on in the acute care setting. You may have the opportunity to work in the ICU or emergency department as a team member under the direction of a registered nurse. You might be required to have additional education and certification in IV therapy as well as ventilator care. While there are acute care settings where LPNs are no longer utilized, there are others who have retained their LPNs and others that are going back to LPNs to bolster their medical teams. As the PracticalNursing.org website indicates (2017), LPNs have the capacity to be flexible and are able to provide a higher level of care to patients beyond the scope of practice of the certified nursing assistant. The LPN can manage the care of the patient under the supervision

© Springer International Publishing AG 2018
C. Kruschke, *Leadership Skills for Licensed Practical Nurses Working with the Aging Population*, https://doi.org/10.1007/978-3-319-69862-5_9

of the registered nurse and provide additional services including medication management and wound care management. Team-based nursing might include the registered nurse, licensed practical nurse, and certified nursing assistants as members of the team, each providing a level of care based on their own scope of practice (Zawora et al, 2015). However, bear in mind hospitals that are magnet status or applying for magnet status tend not to hire LPNs. In the hospital setting, the LPN usually does not hold a leadership or management position.

9.4   The Role of the LPN in the Nursing Home Setting

For most states, the role of the LPN in the long term care setting is similar. In this setting, the LPN is able to take on a leadership role within a specific unit or even at the organizational level. In many long-term care homes, there are more LPNs working in the role of staff nurse than registered nurses (RNs). As reported on the PracticalNursing. org website (2017), LPNs receive a great deal of training including the following:

- Medication administration.
- Wound care.
- Pain management.
- Documentation.
- Data collection.
- Ostomy care.
- Monitor residents for changes in condition.

Licensed practical nurses (LPNs) continue to be trained to be supervised by RNs. LPNs may also be supervised by physicians, advanced practice nurses, and physician assistants. However, as stated previously, in the environment of the nursing home, the LPN can be a manager and a leader (Brandburg, 2012). With this role comes great responsibility. This book has been written to guide you on this path by providing knowledge that will guide you as you continue to gain skills and abilities to be a manager or leader and the attitude to accomplish great things in this new role.

9.5   The Role of the LPN in the Assisted Living Setting

Given the information provided for the role of the LPN in the nursing home setting, we can apply the same information to the role of the LPN in the assisted living setting. In this setting, the LPN can take on additional tasks such as completing data collection to determine if a potential resident will fit the requirements for admission to the assisted living setting. In addition, the LPN can also take on the role of the manager in the assisted living setting (Brandburg, 2012). While the LPN is not specifically trained as a manager in the assisted living setting, with training from the organization, the LPN is capable of carrying out this role successfully.

9.6 The Role of the LPN in the Home Health Setting

The role of the LPN in the home health setting is based on the education of the LPN. While the LPN works under the supervision of a RN, the LPN has the capacity to work independently in the home of specific clients. The LPN can provide care within the scope of practice in each specific state. This includes those same tasks identified earlier and outlined in the client's care plan.

9.7 Role of the LPN as a Nurse Leader

The LPN takes on the role of a nurse leader within the context of the care environment that allows for this to occur. Most often, the LPN would need to work in the nursing home setting or the assisted living setting. With these environments, the LPN would be expected to take on specific traits of a nurse leader as follows:

9.7.1 Walk the Walk and Talk the Talk

This is an important trait of a nurse leader. This particular trait refers to the nurse leader as walking the walk and talking the talk. This means the leader says what is meant and means what is said. This also means the leader backs up what has been said with actions. For example, being totally honest requires you to tell the truth as well as believe in the truth. Your actions must be trustworthy.

9.7.2 Management by Walking Around

This means the nurse leader exhibits one or more traits of a leader and does not hide behind an office desk. Instead the nurse leader makes rounds throughout the shift to make sure to be visible and to share those traits with the entire team:

• Address issues the way you would want them addressed.
• Model the behavior.
• Catch your employees doing something righ.t
• Do not ask others to do tasks you would not do yourself.

Roles of the LPN in the health-care environment:

• Meet with employees and get to know them.
• Employee development.
• Spend time with employees.

9.8   Identify the Role of the LPN in the Delegation Process

9.8.1   Delegation

- Delegation of duties is an integral aspect of the role of the Licensed Practical Nurse (LPN). The LPN is able to delegate duties to another LPN or a certified nursing assistant (CNA). In addition, if the work environment includes Qualified Medication Administration Personnel (QMAPs), the LPN is also able to delegate tasks to QMAPs.
- In order to complete the delegation process effectively, the LPN must know the rules and regulations for CNAs and QMAPs in the state the LPN works in. In addition, the LPN must know the rules and regulations for the LPN related to the ability to delegate tasks including who can delegate and to whom tasks can be delegated (Corazzini, 2010). Chapter 12 provides information regarding the LPN nurse practice act for each state.
- Delegation of tasks requires the LPN to understand the tasks to be delegated and who can actually complete those tasks (Corazzini, 2010). When the LPN delegates tasks, the LPN remains responsible for those tasks which have been delegated to the CNA. This means when you delegate the care of residents to the CNA, you remain accountable for the care each resident receives. This care must meet standards of practice as well as facility policies and procedures. The CNA is also required to provide the care delegated to them based on standards of practice and facility policies and procedures. Failure to follow standards of practice and/or facility policies and procedures is the responsibility of the CNA. When you delegate the care of residents to the CNA, you have a responsibility to oversee the care of the residents and make yourself available to the CNA for questions or concerns related to the care of the residents. You also have a responsibility to ensure the CNA is aware of the care needs of the residents and the CNA has the knowledge, skills and abilities to meet the needs of the residents assigned to a specific CNA.
- The steps you need to take in the delegation process includes:
  - Planning the steps necessary to provide care to all the residents on the unit.
  - Communication of the plan to the appropriate staff members.This step includes delegation (Corazzini, 2010; O'Daniel and Rosenstein, 2013).
  - Supervise and follow-up on the tasks delegated.
  - Evaluate the outcome of care related to the tasks delegated.

- Roles of the nurse/role of the CNA:
  - Use effective communication skills (O'Daniel and Rosenstein, 2013).
  - Prioritize the needs of patients.
  - Direct certified nursing assistants to provide care to residents within their knowledge, skills, and abilities.
  - Supervise and evaluate the care of residents by certified nursing assistants.
  - Assist certified nursing assistants to complete their assigned duties (American Nurses Association and the National Council of State Boards of Nursing, 2006).

9.9   Aspects Integral to Managing the Care Environment

When considering each level of care being provided to elders, we need to consider the following aspects of care that should not be altered.

9.9.1   Quality of Care

Informally, patients talk to each other and reveal the treatment they received or perceive they received from providers. This information is shared with family and friends. If the information is negative, family and friends may seek out another provider if their insurance or payer source allows for the change. If the information is positive, family and friends may seek to receive care from that provider if their insurance or payer source allows for the change. Additionally, consumers are able to compare providers through the Centers for Medicare and Medicaid Services. This is true for hospitals and nursing homes.

9.9.2   Person-Centered Care

In addition to providing quality care, we are also required to provide person-centered care. This means the older adult becomes the center becomes an integral member of the care team. The resident is provided education regarding their medical needs as well as the services offered in the care environment. The older adult then makes decisions regarding which services they will accept and which services they will decline. Remember, older adults have the right to make their own decisions. It is up to you to make sure the older adult has all the information they need to make informed decisions. If the older adult is not able to make their own decisions, you need to consult with the designee for the older adult.

9.9.3   Knowledge, Skills, and Attitudes of Staff

Patients want the provider staff to be knowledgeable, have excellent skills, and have a positive attitude. If any of the staff members are not able to provide any one of the three elements, patients will be less receptive and may not return to the provider. Staff hold a great deal of power when it comes to a provider's ability to attract customers. For example, if you are a patient in the hospital and the caregiver assigned to you is grumpy and comes across as not wanting to provide your care but grudgingly does so, you may report this behavior or you may choose not to use that provider again. When I was having my first child, I went to the not-for-profit hospital where I grew up because it was religious-based. I was very unhappy with the care I received because I was not allowed to hold my daughter while receiving pain medication, not even with staff present. With my subsequent two deliveries, I opted to go to the for-profit hospital. Providers need to make sure staff have the requisite knowledge, skills, and attitude to provide quality care to the patients using the services. This is true regardless of the provider type. Patients have high expectations for the type of care expected. When we fall short of those expectations, the result can be a loss of customers to our competition. The LPN has a significant role ensuring they maintain the highest level of knowledge, skills, and attitude for themselves and their care team. This is a requirement in order to delegate tasks to other staff.

9.9.4   Staffing Structure

Staffing structure is very important in the provision of care. If a provider does not provide adequate staffing, this will impact the ability of the staff to provide quality care. As a patient, how many of us would want to use the services of a provider if the staffing level was inadequate? Providers need to consider this when the staffing structure is being considered and the hours per patient day calculated. The LPN needs to make sure the unit they are overseeing as the nurse has adequate staffing to cover the number of residents on a specific unit including their specific acuity needs.

9.9.5   Cleanliness of the Facility

This factor is very important to consider. Many of us base our decision about a location based on how the environment looks. The theory behind this thinking may be related to our belief that if a provider cannot take care of their own property, how will they take care of their customers? For example, I visited a hospital that was very run down and not kept up well. The waiting room was not clean and much of the furniture was torn. My impression of this hospital was less than stellar. I would not want to use a hospital that is so unkept. I would make other arrangements. If I visit a nursing home and the nursing home has an unhygienic odor, I may opt out of using the facility in the future. As a nursing home administrator and director of nursing, I was adamant that the facility must be clean at all times. Potential customers can come through a facility at any time, and first impressions may be the only opportunity to gain interest from potential customers. One final note, an old medical building can be appealing if it is kept clean and in good repair. As a LPN, you have an important responsibility to ensure your unit is clean and presentable to the residents as well as visitors. If the unit is unkempt, the residents will feel neglected and visitors may also feel the same. Staff members may find it difficult to remain positive if the unit is unclean. You need to set the example by helping to keep the unit neat and clean. When you see something out of place, put it back where it belongs. If there is clutter, eliminate the clutter. Pick up items that do not belong on the floor. Put things away after they have been used. The responsibility of the unit belongs equally to everyone not just housekeeping.

9.9.6   Reputation

Reputation is an important element as well. How do we come across to our customers, staff, peers, and the general public? If we have the reputation for providing quality care, this information will filter to our potential customers. Inversely, if we do not have a good reputation, this will also filter to our potential customers. Many of us decide who will care for us based on reputation. Again, we talk to family and friends to learn who provides their care. We trust family and friends to give us correct information we can use to make our own decision regarding who will provide our care. Reputation is an intrinsic value for a provider. This means the provider is able to apply a dollar value to their reputation, which can only happen if the reputation is positive. Think about the nursing homes or other health care providers who have been in the news. Was the information considered good or bad? Based on what you heard, would you live there? Would you recommend the nursing home or other provider to friends or family? What about the reputation of the staff? If members of the staff are unhappy, how will staff come across to the residents and/or family members? Think about your staff and the steps you can take to support them and provide an atmosphere that is welcoming. Leading by example is an important way to change the atmosphere on your unit and in the entire nursing home. Choose your attitude wisely and model the behavior you expect from your team members.

References

American Nurses Association and the National Council of State Boards of Nursing (2006) Joint statement on delegation. Publisher: Authors

Brandburg G (2012) Nursing roles in health care and long-term care. In: Encyclopedia of health & aging. SAGE, Thousand Oaks, CA, pp 423–425

Corazzini K, Anderson R, Rapp C, Mueller C, McConnell E, Lekan D (2010) Delegation in long-term care: scope of practice or job description? Online J Issues Nurs 15(2):4

O'Daniel M. & Rosenstein A (2013) Chapter 33. Professional communication and team collaboration. Retrieved from https://www.researchgate.net/publication/239591768_Chapter_33_Professional_Communication_and_Team_Collaboration

Practical Nursing.org (2017). Working as a licensed practical nurse (LPN). Retrieved from http://www.practicalnursing.org/working-as-licensed-practical-nurse-lpn

Zawora M, O'Leary C, Bonat J (2015) Turning team-based care into a winning proposition. J Fam Pract 64(3):159–164

Developing a Culture Change Person-Centered Environment

10

10.1 Introduction

"Culture change" is the common name given to the national movement for the transformation of older adult services, based on person-directed values and practices where the voices of elders and those working with them are considered and respected. Core person-directed values are choice, dignity, respect, self-determination, and purposeful living" (Pioneer Network, 2017a, para 2).

10.1.1 Objectives

- Define what culture change is.
- Define person-centered care.
- Identify benefits of culture change.
- Describe steps that can be taken toward culture change.
- Explain approaches to implementing culture change.
- Explore the relationship between culture change and the regulatory climate.
- Describe the role of the LPN in implementing culture change.

10.2 What Is Culture Change?

Culture change is intended to transform the medical model of care to a person-centered model of care through transformation of the mind and spirit. This does not mean we do not meet the medical needs of the individual. We combine the medical model with a model that embraces the human spirit resulting in a more holistic approach to the care of the aging population.

© Springer International Publishing AG 2018
C. Kruschke, *Leadership Skills for Licensed Practical Nurses Working with the Aging Population*, https://doi.org/10.1007/978-3-319-69862-5_10

10.2.1 What is Person-Centered Care?

Person centered care has been identified by the National Nursing Home Quality Improvement Campaign (2017) as the promotion of individualized care developed based on each person's ability to reach their optimum level of physical, psychosocial, and mental well-being. Each individual has the right to make their own choices with purpose and meaning. In turn, each care provider needs to understand the importance of each individual to make their own decisions and to have a life with purpose and meaning.

10.2.2 The Eden Alternative International

The Eden Alternative is an international non-profit organization founded by Dr. William Thomas in response to his belief in providing person-directed care through culture change. He developed the Eden Alternative as a means to transform the living environment of elders to embrace each as an individual. I completed my dissertation based on the Eden Alternative philosophy of care at a nursing home in the Midwest. The findings of this research indicated the Eden Alternative made a difference in the outcomes of the residents who were part of the research I completed. Dr. Thomas believed if the plagues of loneliness, helplessness, and boredom could be alleviated, the lives of elders would be enhanced. From these humble beginnings, the Eden Alternative philosophy has evolved into an international organization continuing to promote quality of life and well-being for elders wherever they live and work. This organization provides education, consultation services and community outreach related to culture change and person-directed care. The Eden Alternative website provides current information regarding the mission, vision and values as well as the ten guiding principles that guide the educators and mentors who promote and advocate for elders nationally and internationally. Additional information can be viewed on the Eden Alternative website at http://www.edenalt.org/

The plagues of loneliness, helplessness, and boredom are important to consider when discussing culture change and person-directed care. While elders may or may not attend activities of their choice, if there are no activities they enjoy, they will eventually succumb to loneliness because they have not had the opportunity to build lasting relationships with their peers or care partners. Human beings also need to feel wanted and needed, providing some type of care to others. This does not necessarily mean hands-on care, but providing care in a variety of ways showing another human being how much they care about them. Without the ability to care for other living beings, the elder will succumb to helplessness. Boredom occurs when elders do not have choices regarding how they would like to spend their day. Doing the same thing every day because there are no other options leads to boredom. We need to provide a community approach in our long-term care homes. The community approach includes a wide variety of individuals including the elders, children, adults, care partners, friends, family, and elders. There also needs to be spontaneity that can only occur when we come together in a variety of ways (Thomas, 1996).

Dr. Thomas relates an experience he had as the Medical Director of a nursing home in the state of New York. He was visiting a woman living at the nursing home. During that visit, she reached out to him and told him how lonely she was. He had no medical intervention that would "heal" her loneliness. It was at this point that he knew he needed to change his approach to the care and the entire health care industry needed to make changes in order to provide the care the elders needed beyond their diagnoses. The Eden Alternative came out of this revelation. Dr. Thomas has worked tirelessly for over 20 years to bring his message to communities across the United States as well as internationally.

The ten principles of the Eden Alternative were developed as the path to improve the lives of elders. These principles can be applied to any environment where elders live. The Ten Principles can be found at the Eden Alternative website, http://www.edenalt.org/about-the-eden-alternative/mission-vision-values/

10.2.3 Pioneer Network

Pioneer Network was founded in 1997 by a group of professionals working in long term care to change the culture of care for elders to a person-centered approach embracing the uniqueness of each individual. The aim of Pioneer Network is "transforming the culture of aging in America" (Pioneer Network, 2017b, para. 1). Pioneer Network has developed a variety of resources to assist organizations and individuals to move away from the medical model of care to a person-centered approach to caring for our elders embracing each elder as an individual. There are a variety of stakeholders who have joined this movement to create a transformation in the culture of care for elders. These stakeholders include:

- Policy makers
- Consumers including elders, family, members and friends
- Educators and researchers
- Providers including organizations and care partners
- Community members

The Pioneer Network founders developed the values and principles continuing to guide this organization. These values and principles can be applied to any environment where the elders live or work. These values and principles can be found at the Pioneer Network website, https://www.pioneernetwork.net/about-us/mission-vision-values/

10.2.4 The Journey towards Culture Change and Person-Centered Care

Regardless of which culture change philosophy or model of care an organization embraces, the journey towards culture change and person-centered care does not end. This is a perpetual journey moving at the speed of life to embrace each individual as an important part of the greater community within and outside of the care home where the elder lives or works. You might be asking yourself how this can be accomplished when there are many patients who must be considered. The answer lies in the belief we can change the outcome for each patient based on an individualized plan of care. This process requires us to embrace each patient as a human being with their own plan for themselves. In culture change this is considered a **growth plan** because we never stop growing or evolving, even if we are no longer able to remain in our own home. We need to embrace growth of individuals as the rule rather than the exception.

10.2.5 Benefits of Culture Change

Culture change and person-centered care is intended to improve the lives of elders living in nursing homes, but has the added benefit of being able to be applied wherever elders live and work. Therefore, culture change and person-centered care improves lives of elders regardless of their location. According to Grabowski et al (2014), culture change has been driven by several innovative care models including the Eden Alternative and the Green House Model. Grabowski pointed to several studies that have shown positive differences between Eden homes and non-Eden homes. Further, the Grabowski study was able to point to Eden homes having fewer health-related deficiencies during the survey process as compared to non-Eden homes. Thus, the potential exists that culture change "may improve nursing home processes of care" (Grabowski et al, 2014, p. S42).

10.2.6 Approaches to Implementing Culture Change

I am sure you are asking yourself if you can implement any changes in your organization and if those changes will be embraced or met with resistance. The first part of the question is a resounding "YES!" you can implement changes within yourself and share what you are doing with your fellow care partners. You just need to start by changing one belief you have held related to the care of the aging population and embrace the new belief. You need to remember this journey is not just about plants, animals, and children; but something deep inside of you that needs to be nourished and moved forward every day. Calling a "bib" a "clothing protector" is not all you can do but it is a starting point.

10.2.7 Culture Change and the Regulatory Climate

We hear many stories for and against culture change based on the regulatory climate. However, those of us who have already started on our culture change journey realize the regulatory climate has shifted, and we are seeing person-centered care move away from a philosophy of care which may or may not be embraced to a culture of care expected to be threaded throughout the organization in a variety of ways to sustain elders and others within an atmosphere embracing each human being.

What has happened over time is a shift away from the medical model of care in the long-term care setting to one embracing culture change and person-centered care.

The State Operations Manual was revised as of March 8, 2017, to include culture change and person-centered care as a regulatory requirement. The terms "person-centered care", "resident's goals", and "preferences" were used multiple times throughout the revised State Operations Manual. This points to the regulatory climate as favoring culture change and person-centered care (Centers for Medicare and Medicaid Services, 2017).

10.2.8 The Role of the LPN in Implementing Culture Change

You have the power to shift your thinking away from the nursing home as an institution and calling it home. Start to use the words meaning home rather than institution. Change starts from the inside out within you and from you.

Know each resident and understanding what their preferences are (Weiner and Ronch, 2014). This information is not limited to the medical needs of each resident, but how each resident wants their care needs met.

The LPN needs to accept the care environment as the resident's home before the resident and other care partners will do the same. Believe the resident is home and share the belief with the resident and other care partners and team members. Knock on the resident's room door before entering every time. After all, this is the resident's home and you would not just walk in the resident's home if the resident lived in a neighborhood environment. Talk about their room as their private space even if they share a room with someone else. Half the room is theirs and they have the right to decide what happens in their space.

You need to look at change from the perspective change will happen, and what is left to decide is when and how change will happen. You need to be part of the team developing the steps to the change including the steps to implementation of the change. Join the team meetings and learn as much as you can. Having this knowledge will prepare you for the change (Weiner and Ronch, 2014).

Slide 10.1: Culture change
Culture change reflects the movement away from the medical model of health care toward a model that is patient-centered. Culture change promotes and advocates for the older adult in the following ways:
- Choice and Self-determination: The older adult should be able to make their own choices. These choices can include the time they want to get up in the morning, when they want to eat and what they want to eat, and the care they will receive, to name a few. The older adult also has the right to determine their future goals and develop the plan to meet those goals.
- Respect and Dignity: All older adults deserve to be treated with respect and dignity. Older adults retain their right to be treated with respect and dignity regardless of where they live. Remember, older adults are not children.

References

Centers for Medicare and Medicaid Services (2017) State operations manual. Appendix PP
    –Guidance to surveyors for long term care facilities. Retrieved from https://www.cms.gov/
    Regulations-and-Guidance/Guidance/Manuals/downloads/som107ap_pp_guidelines_ltcf.pdf
Grabowski D, O'Malley A, Afendulis C, Caudry D, Elliot A, Zimmerman S (2014) Culture change
    and nursing home quality of care. Gerontologist 54(S1):S35–S45
National Nursing Home Quality Improvement Campaign (2017) Person-centered care. Retrieved
    from https://www.nhqualitycampaign.org/goalDetail.aspx?g=PCC
Pioneer Network (2017a) What is culture change? Retrieved from https://www.pioneernetwork.
    net/culture-change/what-is-culture-change/
Pioneer Network (2017b) Our vision and mission. Retrieved from https://www.pioneernetwork.
    net/about-us/mission-vision-values/
Thomas W (1996) Life worth living. Vanderwyck and Burnham, Acton, MA
Weiner A, Ronch J (2014) Models and pathways for person-centered elder care. Health Professions
    Press, Baltimore, MD

Suggested Reading

Eden Alternative (2017) The Eden Alternative domains of well-being. Retrieved from http://www.
    edenalt.org/about-the-eden-alternative/the-eden-alternative-domains-of-well-being/

Current and Future Trends in Long-Term Care

11

11.1 Introduction: Where It All Began

The long-term care industry first developed in response to the need for efficiency and economy of scale for those needing health care beyond the acute care setting and those providing the care. Long-term care facilities began as poor houses and religious care homes in response to the need for care of the elderly and infirm. Following the addition of Medicare and Medicaid as payer sources, the long-term care industry exploded. Anyone could start a nursing home if they had the money and the building to house the patients. Nursing homes were first developed to replicate the acute care setting and were often attached to the acute care setting with physicians as the administrators. As for-profit entities entered the long-term care arena, the nursing home became freestanding and without the medical connection to a specific hospital or physician group. The development of assisted living facilities provided another avenue to break into the long-term care market and make an even greater profit than was realized in the nursing home setting. With the majority of assisted living facilities only private-pay, the profit margins grew, creating an environment of growth and expansion.

We have learned how far health care has come in the care of the aging population. In this chapter we look at the trends that are occurring today and what tomorrow will bring.

11.2 Objectives

- Identify the current health-care trends in the care of the aging population.
- Anticipate the future trends in the care of the aging population.
- Explore the role of the licensed practical nurse as a leader today and tomorrow.

© Springer International Publishing AG 2018
C. Kruschke, *Leadership Skills for Licensed Practical Nurses Working
with the Aging Population*, https://doi.org/10.1007/978-3-319-69862-5_11

11.3   What We Have Learned

We continue to live in exiting times as the care of the aging population continues to evolve away from the medical model of nursing care for the aging population to one that now embraces the whole person through the impetus of culture change. We see the value of person-centered care that places the elder in the center of the care team. As we continue the journey toward person-directed care where the elder is the director of their own care, we anticipate the future knowing that each step we take in this direction will provide the tools we need to provide quality care to our aging population.

You are at the forefront of this journey as you lead the changes taking place on your unit and within your organization and as part of a national and international effort to provide the best care possible to your residents/patients/clients. Moving forward requires us to look back retrospectively to learn from our past regarding the care of the aging population.

We know nursing homes were set up to look like hospitals because that is what we knew. We learned through the culture change movement that nursing homes need to be set up **as homes for the aging population**. We may not be able to change the brick and mortar in all cases, but we can change the appearance of nursing homes to look less like a hospital and more like a home. Chapter 10 provided a view of this belief.

A variety of **payment programs** have been developed by the federal government through the Centers for Medicare and Medicaid Services to meet the financial needs of older adults who require payment assistance to meet their health-care needs in the long run (Centers for Medicare and Medicaid Services, 2017). However, through these systems, reimbursement has not been equitable and many older adults are not able to live in the least restrictive environment because they do not have the funds to pay for those services. For example, wanting to live in an assisted living home might be the ideal situation, but, if the funding is not available, that individual could end up living in a nursing home instead. Allowing the funding for each older adult to follow that adult regardless of where they choose to reside as long as they meet the criteria for that level of services. Thus, if someone wants to live in an assisted living home rather than a nursing home, the funding would be available to make that decision.

Home health is important because many elderly would rather live at home and have caregivers come to them (Bodie, 2015). Increasing funding for home health will keep more elderly in their own homes. Additionally, as discussed in the previous paragraph, if funding follows the older adult, there would be funding available for that individual to remain in their home as long as there are services available for that individual.

We have developed a variety of **care programs and philosophies** to meet the needs of our aging population. We need to continue developing these programs to ensure older adults remain as independent as possible. This requires us to look beyond the medical needs of each older adult and embrace the entire person, meeting all their needs. We also need to continue advancing education to ensure caregivers understand best practices in relationship to the care of the aging population.

Culture change has shifted our thinking beyond the medical model of care provision to one that is certainly more holistic. We need to honor older adults by asking them what they want rather than telling them what they want. We must abide by their decisions and help them to have the best life possible. Our aging population does not enter the long-term care system to die but to live their best life. This requires us to show respect for older adults, honor their choices, and continue to work with them to maintain a dignified life that includes self-determination (Pioneer Network, 2017b).

11.4   Long-Term Care Today

Long-term care facilities provide **long-term care services** to a variety of individuals. Usually long-term care is associated with providing care to older adults. The current trend has included individuals under the age of 65 who need long-term care services. Long-term care continues to include a variety of providers offering different levels of services. While we learned about these care environments previously, we will review those care environments here.

Nursing homes were developed to meet the needs of a growing aging population no longer able to care for themselves. This need resulted in the development of care homes in order to achieve economies of scale in terms of care providers. With older adults in one location, the provision of care became more efficient and effective from the perspective of cost. Additionally, with our resources becoming scarcer including funding and human resources, nursing homes as well as other care environments will become even more important in order to ensure there are enough scarce resources to meet the needs of more of the population (Watson, 2012).

With the introduction of **assisted living homes**, patients needing intermediate nursing care were discharged from nursing homes to assisted living if they were able to pay for the services themselves. Assisted living homes provide a variety of services depending on the needs of the patients, who are often called residents. Services include meal preparation, housekeeping services, laundry services, and medication assistance. Determination of care limitations is based on the licensing requirements in each state (Wilson, 2007).

Residential care apartment complexes provide a variety of services to individuals residing in the complex based on the individual's specific needs. Services can include meal preparation, housekeeping services, laundry services, and/or assistance with activities of daily living (Ajack, n.d.). This is considered an assisted living environment where the individuals live in their own apartments.

Independent living environments include private homes, apartments, and retirement communities. Services in homes and private apartments can be contracted privately with private funds. If an individual requires home health or hospice services, funding can include private funding, private health insurance, and government funding (Senior Care Advice, 2018).

Historically, **home care** has been part of society for centuries as individuals were cared for in their homes by midwives, faith healers, and physicians. The home care industry can trace its roots back to the late 1800s as individuals without funds needed care and society began to find ways to meet care needs in the home. From the beginning the focus has been on the care needs of individuals with an emphasis on keeping individuals in their homes whenever possible. As the cost of care in the hospital rose during the mid-1900s, the call for more home health care was answered by the government by allowing Medicare to pay for home health care (Penn Nursing Science, n.d.).

The **medical home model of care** is emerging as an important alternative in the provision of care for the older adult. This model is led by a physician who coordinates care of the patient with a team of professionals including nurses, therapists, nutritionists, social workers, and others. The Affordable Care Act has provisions supporting this model of care and most states have some type of policy that supports this model of care (National Conference of State Legislatures, 2018).

11.5   Current Trends in the Care Environment

As we have moved from the medical model of care to a culture change environment, we have also looked at quality improvement across the health-care continuum. The nursing home setting is an excellent example of positive trending related to key outcomes identified by the Centers for Medicare and Medicaid Services as important to improve. Safety for residents and staff is important in the medical community and no less important in the nursing home setting.

One of the safety areas of importance requires nursing homes to be **free from chemical** (medication that alters elderly thought processes) **and physical restraints**. A restraint-free environment in health care means that we are consistently avoiding the use of chemical or physical restraints whenever possible in favor of alternative approaches (Centers for Medicare and Medicaid Services, 2017b). A restraint-free environment is an important practice in the provision of patient-centered care.

Reduction in falls is an important safety initiative for residents living in long-term care homes. Falls continue to be a critical issue in the health and well-being of older adults. In addition to the myriad physical, psychological, and emotional ramifications of a fall, there are also financial consequences that must be taken into consideration. Falls can significantly impact the older adult's entire family and causes individuals and families alike to make serious and costly decisions involving their health care, financial options, and living situations, among other decisions (Kruschke, 2016; Kruschke, 2017).

The next area to consider is not consistently considered a safety issue but is considered an important issue for residents living in long-term care homes (Joosse, L. 2011). There needs to be a **reduction in noise** produced by staff especially during the night. Residents have reported staff making noise with equipment and their own voices during the night as care is provided to older adults needing assistance. This can be very distressing to those who are trying to sleep. Sleep deprivation can have a detrimental impact on an older adult's physical and mental well-being. The recommendation is to curb noise especially during the night to allow residents to have a restful sleep. Overhead paging is another concern especially in long-term care homes on the culture change journey. Overhead paging is very noisy. Living in our own homes, we do not use overhead paging and the same needs to apply in long term care homes. There are nursing homes now using cell phones and text messaging to reach our staff and care partners, which is far less intrusive than overhead paging.

Disaster preparedness to ensure elderly is safe even if a catastrophe occurs such as power outages or flooding. Developing an understanding of emergency planning is important to the safety and welfare of patients, staff, and community members (National Consumer Voice, 2016). This is critical especially with the number of natural disasters that occur across the country throughout the year. This year we are reminded of how extreme the weather can be as Texas faced Hurricane Harvey and the devastation we have witnessed including homes older adults ending up with extensive flooding resulting in the forced evacuation of the older adults in these homes. We cannot forget the image of women sitting in wheelchairs in waist-deep water waiting to be rescued. This type of catastrophe plays out far too often. Disaster preparedness helps us to reach out to older adults to set up alternative locations for our elderly population to be moved to when disaster strikes.

The rising cost of technology is another safety concern as long-term care homes look to the advances in technology to improve the care of older adults living in long-term care homes. The rising cost, including the cost of supplies and equipment, can be difficult to offset especially given the limitations in reimbursement to long-term care homes. Another aspect of the cost of technology that needs to be considered is the cost for specialized expertise to operate or utilize the technology.

11.6 Payment Systems

We discussed payment systems and the changes that have taken place through the years since the inception of Medicare and Medicaid. A brief review is beneficial as we discuss the current and future trends in long-term care.

Medicare is intended for individuals over the age of 65, under age 65 with specific disabilities, and individuals with end-stage renal disease (ESRD). This coverage includes hospital care, medical care provided in clinics by physicians, and nursing home coverage for short periods of time. Additional services covered include durable medical equipment, ambulance services, some medications, and home health care (Medicare.gov, 2017). **Medicaid** is financed by the federal government as well as each state under a joint agreement. The federal government reimburses each state for their Medicaid program based on predetermined criteria such as per capita income (Medicare.gov, 2017).

Private insurance is a voluntary program. For the older adult, private insurance is generally purchased through a private insurance company as a Medicare supplement policy. Private insurance premiums are determined by the insurance company based on actuary tables that review a variety of variables. Insured individuals may be required to pay co-pays and/or deductibles determined by the private insurance company. **Capitation** provides payments to health-care providers based on the number of patients covered by the insurer. The rate of payment is negotiated between the capitation provider and the health-care provider (Senior Care Advice, 2018).

Veteran's benefits are provided to military personnel while they are in the service as well as after they leave the service. There are over 12 million veterans over the age of 65. Benefits include:

- Disability
- Pension
- Education and training
- Health care
- Home loans
- Insurance
- Burial (U.S. Department of Veterans Affairs, 2017)

Private pay is intended to refer to patients who pay for their health care out-of-pocket. Patients may pay privately for certain services not covered by their health insurance plan, co-payments, deductibles, or the cost associated with using a provider outside their health insurance plan. Co-payments are usually due at the time the service is provided. Today, it is rarer for older adults to pay privately for nursing home services. Patients in assisted living still tend to pay privately. If a private pay patient is admitted to the nursing home setting, the chances are greater that the individual does not have a payer source including the lack of private funds.

11.7   Reimbursement Alternatives

Reimbursement alternatives have been discussed but will be reviewed here as part of our discussion related to current and future trends in long-term care.

The goal of the **prospective payment system** is to motivate health-care providers to deliver services in the most cost-effective manner possible while providing quality care. The payment structure takes into consideration the diagnoses of the patients and the usual and customary care necessary for that diagnosis. The government oversees the prospective payment system (Centers for Medicare and Medicaid Services, 2017a). **Diagnostic-related groups (DRGs)** are used in the acute care setting and home health to determine the reimbursement rate for provider (Centers for Medicare and Medicaid Services, 2017c). The provider is given a fixed amount of dollars for each DRG. If the provider is able to reduce cost and save money, the provider reaps the benefit of this savings as the payment remains the same. Conversely, if the provider spends more than what is reimbursed, the provider must absorb those costs. **Resource utilization groups (RUGs)** are used in the long-term care setting to determine the reimbursement rate for providers (Centers for Medicare and Medicaid Services, 2017d). The payment structure is similar to DRGs. The RUGs are initially assigned at the time the first Minimum Data Set (MDS) is completed for each resident admitted to the nursing home setting. While the resident resides in the nursing home, the MDS will be completed at specific intervals and, with each MDS completed, a new RUGs score will be assigned. This RUGs score is the basis for reimbursement to the nursing home based on the care needs of each older adult. **Resource-based relative value units (RVUs)** are used to determine the reimbursement for physician services provided (Centers for Medicare and Medicaid Services, 2017e). The RVU is usually considered as an increment of time, such as 10 min or 15 min. The value of the physician's services is determined by using the resource-based relative value unit scale.

11.8   Reimbursement System Changes

The federal government continues to strive to reduce overall costs for the care of the aging population. In order to reduce costs, the Centers for Medicare and Medicaid Services has developed a variety of programs that are intended to reduce cost and provide incentives for nursing homes to meet specific outcome requirements.

11.8.1 Pay for Performance

Pay for performance is an incentive program providing funds to nursing homes that meet and/or exceed specific quality requirements based on quality indicators monitored by the Centers for Medicare and Medicaid as part of the current reimbursement system. Hospitals and physicians also receive incentives to improve patient outcomes. There are currently over 180 such programs across the globe. More than half the states have some type of pay for performance program. Review the requirements for your state to determine if this program is offered. Many of the programs have proven to show moderate success in following through on initiatives to improve the patient experience. Program goals include more efficient management of resources, promoting medical practices that provide a safe environment for patients and following evidence-based practice in the provision of care (Health Affairs, 2012).

11.8.2 Payment Bundling

Payment bundling is another incentive program developed by the government and initiated January, 2013. This payment structure provides a lump-sum payment for services provided to a patient by multiple providers. For example, if an older adult is admitted to the hospital for a fractured hip, the reimbursement is based on the cost of care by the interdisciplinary team. There is one payment made to the hospital with the intent of paying for all the services provided while the older adult was in the hospital. This program is intended to avoid duplication of services. Another anticipated goal of this program is avoiding complications by having providers work together rather than working in silos. Currently the bundling of payments is voluntary. We anticipate seeing this program expand and become mandatory at some point in the future (Senior Care Advice, 2018).

11.8.3 Never Events

Never events were name for those outcomes the Centers for Medicare and Medicaid deemed should never have happened or considered avoidable. If the outcome is considered avoidable, CMS reduces or eliminates reimbursement for that event. For example, if a resident develops a pressure wound in the hospital, the cost to treat the wound will not be reimbursed. Additional outcomes that are considered never events include infections, falls, deaths not considered natural, or abuse of an elderly person (Centers for Medicare and Medicaid Services, 2008).

11.8.4 Thirty-Day Readmissions

The Centers for Medicare and Medicaid Services (2017f) oversees the 30-day readmission program which is intended to reduce the number of readmissions to the hospital setting for the same diagnosis as the original admission. Readmission diagnoses covered under this policy include myocardial infarction, heart failure, and pneumonia. If a hospital experiences excessive readmissions within 30 days for the same patient with the same diagnosis, the hospital's reimbursement rate is reduced.

11.9   Future Trends

We have reviewed the current trends related to the long-term care setting. In this section we will look at the anticipated future trends.

11.9.1 Better Integration of Services and Financing

Long-term care integration of services include the integration of home care, community-based long-term care services, primary care services, acute care services, and institutional care services (nursing home, assisted living). Integration of services also includes behavioral health partnerships with state aging agencies. **Accountable care organizations (ACOs)** are groups of providers who agree to provide care to a specific group of older adults for a specific fee for all services provided (Senior Care Advice, 2018). We are already learning about ACOs and anticipate a growth in this service system. **Aging and Disability Resource Centers** are single points of entry to the health-care system for older adults (Administration for Community Living, 2017). This service allows the older adult to enter the system at one point for all services needed rather than having to enter at multiple points depending on the service required. **Person-centered medical homes** provide an integration/coordination of care between health-care professionals, social services, and the patient's family. Often this care is provided in the patient's home. Another example of a person-centered medical home is a primary care physician's clinical practice (Agency for Healthcare Research and Quality (AHRQ), 2017).

11.10 Increased Accountability to Health-Care Consumers

Consumers are no longer willing to accept the status quo related to the health care they receive. When I first became a nurse, the elderly we cared for accepted the care system they became part of when they entered the nursing home setting. The medical model of care is what they had received in the hospital and it seemed to make sense to them. However, as we have moved away from the medical model to a culture change model, the aging population is no longer willing to go back to the old system. As our generations have aged, it is the baby boomers who are expected to enter the long-term care system in the future. The baby boomers have a completely different mind-set and the providers of care need to be prepared for this unique generation.

The government also has high expectations and has initiated programs to hold providers accountable for the care provided. As discussed previously, programs have been developed to improve outcomes while saving money overall. Accountability includes the following.

11.10.1 Use of Fewer Resources Efficiently

When we consider resources in the provision of health care, resources include:

- *Financial*: Health-care providers need to educate their employees regarding the importance of using scarce resources more efficiently and effectively. When considering financial resources, providers need to be fiscally responsible.
- *Human resources*: When we consider human resources, we need to consider how we staff our health-care facilities. For example, we need to provide the right amount of staff to meet the needs of our patients
- *Equipment and supplies*: Use only the supplies needed.
- *Health-care resources*: Health care has a finite level of resources that can be used at any given time. Use these resources wisely (Fraser, Encinosa and Glied, 2008; Resnik, 2007).

11.10.2 Increased Innovation and Diversity in the Provision of Health-Care Services

Diversity is important in the provision of health care as our society becomes more diverse from the perspective of the patients/residents/clients as well as those who are part of the care team. We need to provide culturally competent care that meets the needs of this diverse population. A more inclusive definition of health is required in order to embrace everyone in the health-care system (Institute for Healthcare Improvement, 2013). Marginalized populations are especially vulnerable including the elderly, underinsured and uninsured. While we considered the Affordable Care Act as the answer to the issues within our health-care system, given the issues currently being faced related to this legislation, we will need to look to the future for answers.

Innovation in health care includes new products, services, and programs to meet the diverse needs of the population accessing health care including the older adult.

11.10.3   Less Focus on Treatment and More Focus on Education, Prevention, and Care Management

The medical model of health care focuses on treatment of diseases and the disease process while the person-directed care model focuses on education, prevention, and care management. Initially, nursing homes were built to look like hospitals with a central nursing station and long hallways. The focus was on the disease process and not the elderly person. The nursing home sets the rules and everyone followed them. Currently we are moving toward the culture change model with a focus on person-centered care with a focus on education, prevention, and care management, which meets the objectives of Healthy People 2020 (HealthyPeople.gov, 2014). Long hallways are giving way to an environment where care providers focus on the individual.

11.10.4   Increased Use of Data Collection and Analysis

Data collection and analysis is growing across the health-care continuum including long-term care. We are hearing more about big data and the ability to "data mine" using these large data sets as we research outcomes to determine evidence-based practice (American Health Information Management Association, 2012). We know that big data analysis has the capacity to change and improve our system of health care by adding to the body of knowledge that leads to evidence-based practice. Additionally, the use of data collection and analysis helps us to develop national standards as benchmarks for providers to compare with.

11.10.5   Movement Toward Improvement of Population Health

We need to integrate primary care and public health in order to improve population health. We need to develop a plan to better understand the issues facing our older adults as well as our entire population. The primary goal is to improve population health with the underlying goal of reducing disparity in health care between those who receive care and those who do not. Population health focuses on health services, quality of life, and injury prevention when we consider the older adult

(HealthyPeople.gov, 2014; and Kindig and Stoddart, 2003; Population Health Alliance, 2017).

11.11 Culture Change

As we have learned, we need to develop a plan of action to incorporate culture change into a work environment in the promotion of quality care to the older adult. This includes finding alternative trends in senior housing that will provide additional opportunities for our aging population to live their best life in the environment of their choosing.

11.12 New Trends in Senior Housing

11.12.1 Home Care

Our demographics speak to the growth in our aging population and the desire of most individuals to age in place in their own homes. This will result in a growth in home care to accommodate the additional individuals who require some type of support to remain in their own homes. This growth is also spurred by economic pressure to reduce costs especially related to our aging population. Community support will be essential to ensure there are enough services to meet the ongoing and growing demand.

11.12.2 Villages

For many of us, living in "villages" was never part of our plan when considering our options to age in place. However, this choice makes sense for those of us who wish to live among our peers. Using homes in the same neighborhood or apartment homes in the same apartment building provide this "village" atmosphere. It is here the elders come together to organize and coordinate services with an annual or monthly fee to pay for those coordinated services (The Oxford Institute of Population Aging, 2017). This type of environment might be compared to homeowners who pay an HOA fee.

11.12.3 Naturally Occurring Retirement Communities

Naturally occurring retirement communities occur where there are a high number of older adults living in the same geographic area (Masotti et al, 2006). Examples include apartment complexes and retirement communities. Within this geographic area, community support is developed based on the needs and preferences of those living in the retirement community. Consider apartment complexes or private neighborhoods that support the retirement community over the age of 55 or 62 as naturally occurring retirement communities. These communities can also occur by chance as smaller communities are developed and naturally become small retirement communities. I currently live in a neighborhood that has evolved into a natural retirement community with the majority of the neighbors at or beyond retirement age.

11.12.4   Neighborhood-Based Care Home Model

The neighborhood-based care home model engages the entire household as a community helping and supporting each other to remain independent. This household occurs in neighborhoods as older adults come together and live in the same home. Each individual or couple have their own space as well as congregate living spaces to share with the other members of the household. This model is similar to an assisted living home but remains unique because each individual or couple pay rent to the household and remain totally independent. The group may engage a household staffing model by hiring outside support such as a cleaning service or meal preparation with each member of the household paying for part of the service (The Guardian, 2015).

11.13   Growth of Programs to Meet the Needs of the Aging Population

As our population ages, we need to continue growing programs to meet the unique needs of our aging population. The following are programs to meet the needs of the aging population.

11.13.1   PACE Program

The Programs for All-inclusive Care for the Elderly (PACE) is an optional program under Medicare and Medicaid for individuals who are aged 55 and older with chronic care needs (Medicaid.gov, 2017; Medicare.gov, 2017). To participate in the PACE program, individuals must be certified as needing nursing home placement but are able to live safely in the community with PACE services. While an individual might need hospital care or nursing home care, the goal is to remain in the community.

The PACE program has its roots as the On Lok program that was begun in San Francisco serving the older adult community. The intent of this program was to provide services to the older adult by receiving a set payment per older adult per day. The goal of the PACE program continues to embody the belief that older adults with chronic conditions can receive all required care while living in the community.

11.13.2   Nurses Improving Care to Older Adults (NICHE)

The NICHE program is intended to provide quality care to patients over the age of 65 (NICHE, 2017). There are two models of care associated with the NICHE program.

- *Geriatric resource nurse* (*GRN*): This is actually an education and clinical model that focuses on educating the bedside nurse to the special needs of the older adult. The Geriatric resource nurse receives training from an advanced practice nurse to assess and respond to geriatric syndromes in the older adult.
- *Acute Care of the Elderly Medical-Surgical Unit* (*ACE Unit*): The Acute Care of the Elderly Medical-Surgical Unit (ACE Unit) is a dedicated unit specifically geared to the special needs of the older adult (NICHE, 2017, para 2 and para 6).

11.13.3   Advancing Care Excellence for Seniors (ACES)

The goal of ACES is to provide education to nurses that will improve the care of the older adult. Topics include:

- Aging that is individualized
- The complexity of care related to the older adult especially based on comorbidities
- Transitions of care
- Alzheimer's related issues (NICHE, 2017)

11.13.4   Guided Care

Guided Care is a model of care that results in the provision of care that will meet the complex needs of patients with comorbidities. This model of care was developed at Johns Hopkins University in response to the aging older adult population. Guided Care has been found to result in overall satisfaction with the care provided by caregivers as well as the care received by the older adult (John Hopkins Bloomberg School of Public Health, 2013).

11.13.5   Medical Home Model of Care

The medical home model of care is emerging as an important alternative in the provision of care for the older adult. This model is a patient-centered care model led by a physician who coordinates care of the patient with a team of professionals including nurses, therapists, nutritionists, social workers, and others who ensure integration of services at reduced cost. The Affordable Care Act has provisions supporting this model of care and most states have some type of policy that supports this model of care (National Conference of State Legislatures, 2012; Patient-Centered Primary Care Collaborative, 2017).

11.13.6   Transitional Care Models

This program is geared to the older adult with comorbidities including at least five chronic conditions. This model is an evidence-based solution to the challenges related to comorbidities. Transitional care models have shown positive outcomes in the area of avoidance of hospital readmissions, improved health outcomes, and an enhanced care experience as reported by patients and families. Transitional care models are also important in the care for the cognitively impaired (Coalition for Evidence-Based Policy, 2015).

11.14   Growth of Culture Change Care Philosophies

Culture change care philosophies continue to grow as our nation has embraced person-centered care as the preferred model of care. Regulatory bodies have also embraced culture change and person-centered care as the preferred model of care. With this acceptance, person-centered care is growing nationally and internationally in the provision of care for all populations especially our aging population (Pioneer Network, 2017a; Evans, 2017).

11.14.1   Eden Alternative

The Eden Alternative is an alternative philosophy of care that places the resident in the center of the care model. Decisions are made as close to the resident as possible based on patient-directed care. Meeting the unmet needs of the older adult is a vital component of the Eden Alternative.

11.14.2   Pioneer Network

The Pioneer Network is a national not-for-profit organization dedicated to the creation of a culture where elders have a voice, their voices are heard, and their voices are respected. Pioneer Network advocates for person-directed care not system-directed (Pioneer Network, 2017a; Evans, 2017).

11.14.3   Green House Model

Homes that are newly developed providing care to 10–12 residents in a model that shares resources and believes in patient-centered care (The Green House Project, 2018). This model is intended to take the place of nursing homes wherever possible.

This model is similar to an assisted living home where each resident has their own room and bathroom connected to common living areas, but without the long hallways that were the hallmark of nursing homes and early assisted living homes. The Green House model provides the opportunity for older adults to have a meaningful life in homes rather than institutions. In these homes, staff are empowered with mutual respect for each other and the residents living in these homes. Green Houses receive funding from grants and community programs (The Green House Project, 2018).

11.15 Setting the Stage for the Future

We have reviewed the programs and services currently available for the aging population. Now, we will look at how the licensed practical nurse (LPN) can set the stage for the future. The LPN is an important leader in the long-term care setting. For many nursing homes across the United States, the role of the LPN is important to the overall nursing care of our aging population. According to labor statistics, 5% of the RNs working in the United States work in nursing homes. With 2.8 million RNs working in nursing in 2014, this equates to 125,000 RNs working in nursing homes (Bureau of Labor Statistics 2015a). For the licensed practical nurse, there are 719,900 LPNs working in 2014 with 29% work in nursing homes which represents 208,771 LPNs working in the nursing home setting (Bureau of Labor Statistics 2015b).

Each nurse must continue to learn and grow in their role regardless of where they work. This is even more important for LPNs in the long-term care field because of the leadership role the LPN takes on when working in the long-term care setting. The LPN needs to fully understand the LPN scope of practice and to continue working within that scope of practice. The LPN needs to use the values of attitude, trust, and influence to affect change from the medical model of nursing to a culture change person-centered care model of nursing. In addition, the LPN needs to understand the current long-term care environment as well as the trends for the future in order to promote the best quality care possible for the aging population. LPNs are in position to influence the future and must be part of the planning process. This book has strived to provide the information necessary for the LPN to take on this leadership role today and in preparation for tomorrow.

In the words of Dylan Thomas,

Do not go gentle into that good night,Old age should burn and rave at close of day;Rage, rage against the dying of the light.

References

Administration for Community Living (2017) Aging and disability resource centers. Retrieved from https://www.acl.gov/programs/aging-and-disabilitynetworks/aging-and-disability-resource-centers

Agency for Healthcare Research and Quality (AHRQ) (2017) Defining the PCMH. Retrieved from https://pcmh.ahrq.gov/page/defining-pcmh

Ajack K (n.d.) Residential care apartment. Retrieved from https://seniorresourcesonline.com/provider-category/residentialcare-apartment-complexes/

American Health Information Management Association (2012) Data quality management model (updated). Retrieved from http://library.ahima.org/xpedio/groups/public/documents/ahima/bok1_049664.hcsp?dDocName=bok1_049664 ports/olderam/oldam1.html

Bodie A (2015) The growing importance of home health care services. Retrieved from https://www.assisted1.com/growningneedforhomehealthcare/

Bureau of Labor Statistics (2015a) Registered nurses. Retrieved from https://www.bls.gov/ooh/healthcare/registered-nurses.htm#tab-1

Bureau of Labor Statistics (2015b) Licensed Practical and licensed vocational nurses. Retrieved from https://www.bls.gov/ooh/healthcare/licensed-practical-andlicensed-vocational-nurses.htm#tab-3

Centers for Medicare and Medicaid Services (2008) Medicare and medicaid move aggressively to encourage greater patient safety in hospitals and reduce never events. Retrieved from https://www.cms.gov/Newsroom/MediaReleaseDatabase/Press-Releases/2008-Press-Releases-Items/2008-07-313.html

Centers for Medicare and Medicaid Services (2017a) Prospective payment systems. Retrieved from https://www.cms.gov/Medicare/Medicare-Feefor-Service-Payment/ProspMedicareFeeSvcPmtGen/index.html

Centers for Medicare and Medicaid Services (2017b) State operations manual. Retrieved from https://www.cms.gov/Regulations-and-Guidance/Legislation/CFCsAndCoPs/Downloads/som107ap_pp_guidelines_ltcf.pdf

Centers for Medicare and Medicaid Services (2017c) Acute inpatient PPS. Retrieved from https://www.cms.gov/Medicare/Medicare-Fee-for-Service-Payment/AcuteInpatientPPS/index.html

Centers for Medicare and Medicaid Services (2017d) Skilled nursing facility PPS. Retrieved from https://www.cms.gov/Medicare/Medicare-Fee-for-Service-Payment/SNFPPS/index.html

Centers for Medicare and Medicaid Services (2017e) Physician fee schedule. Retrieved from https://www.cms.gov/Medicare/Medicare-Fee-for-Service-Payment/PhysicianFeeSched/index.html

Centers for Medicare and Medicaid Services (2017f) Readmissions reduction program (HRRP). Retrieved from https://www.cms.gov/Medicare/Medicare-Fee-for-Service-Payment/AcuteInpatientPPS/Readmissions-Reduction-Program.html

Coalition for Evidence-Based Policy (2015) Transitional are model – top tier. Retrieved from http://evidencebasedprograms.org/1366-2/transitionalcare-model-top-tier

Evans J (2017) Person-centered care and culture change. Caring for the Ages 18(8):6

Fraser I, Encinosa W, Glied S (2008) Improving efficiency and value in health care: introduction. Health Serv Res 43(5 Pt 2):1781–1786

Health Affairs (2012) Pay-for-performance. Retrieved from http://www.healthaffairs.org/health-policybriefs/brief.php?brief_id=78

HealthyPeople.gov (2014) Educational and community-based programs. Retrieved from https://www.healthypeople.gov/2020/topicsobjectives/topic/educational-and-community-based-programs

Institute for Healthcare Improvement (2013) Diversity and inclusion. Retrieved from http://www.ihi.org/communities/blogs/_layouts/15/ihi/community/blog/itemview.aspx?List=7d1126ec-8f63-4a3b-9926-c44ea3036813&ID=34

John Hopkins Bloomberg School of Public Health (2013) Guided Care. Comprehensive primary care for complex patients. Retrieved from http://guidedcare.org/about-us.asp

Joosse L (2011) Sound levels in nursing homes. J Gerontol Nurs 37(8):30–35

Kindig D, Stoddart G (2003) What is population health? Am J Public Health 93(3):380–383

Kruschke C (2016) Fall prevention in older adults. The University of Iowa. College of Nursing. Barbara and Richard Csomay Center for Gerontological Excellence

Kruschke C (2017) Evidence-based practice guideline: fall prevention for older adults. J Gerontol Nurs 43(11):15–21

Masotti P, Fick R, Johnson-Masotti A, MacLeod S (2006) Healthy naturally occurring retirement communities: a low-cost approach to facilitating healthy aging. Am J Public Health 96(7):1164–1170

Medicaid.gov (2017) Program of all-inclusive care for the elderly. Retrieved from https://www.medicaid.gov/medicaid/ltss/pace/index.html

Medicare.gov (2017) PACE. Retrieved from https://www.medicare.gov/your-medicare-costs/help-paying-costs/pace/pace.html

National Conference of State Legislatures (2012) The medical home model of care. Retrieved from http://www.ncsl.org/research/health/the-medicalhome-model-of-care.aspx

National Conference of State Legislatures (2018) The medical home model of care. Retrieved from http://www.ncsl.org/research/health/the-medicalhome-model-of-care.aspx

National Consumer Voice (2016) Emergency preparedness. Retrieved from http://ltcombudsman.org/issues/emergency-preparedness

NICHE (2017) Program overview. Retrieved from http://www.nicheprogram.org/program-overview/

Patient-Centered Primary Care Collaborative (2017) Defining the medical home. Retrieved from https://www.pcpcc.org/about/medical-home

Penn Nursing Science (n.d.) Home care. Retrieved from https://www.nursing.upenn.edu/nhhc/home-care/

Pioneer Network (2017a) Defining culture change. Retrieved from https://www.pioneernetwork.net/culture-change/what-is-culture-change/

Pioneer Network (2017b) Our vision and mission. Retrieved from https://www.pioneernetwork.net/about-us/mission-vision-values/

Population Health Alliance (2017) Understanding population health. Retrieved from http://populationhealthalliance.org/research/understanding-population-health.html

Resnik D (2007) Responsibility for health: personal, social and environmental. J Med Ethics 33(8):444–445

Senior Care Advice (2018) Independent living. Retrieved from https://seniorcareadvice.com/housing-care/independent-living

The Green House Project (2018) Discover. Retrieved from http://www.thegreenhouseproject.org/about/discover

The Guardian (2015) Cohousing: it makes sense for people with thintogether. Retrieved from https://www.theguardian.com/society/2015/feb/16/cohousing-people-things-common-live-together-older-people gs in common to love

The Oxford Institute of Population Aging (2017) It takes a (retirement) village: how to address the crisis in housing for the elderly. Retrieved from https://www.ageing.ox.ac.uk/blog/it-takes-a-village

U.S. Department of Veterans Affairs (2017) Access and quality in VA health. Retrieved from http://www.accesstocare.va.gov/

Watson S (2012) From almshouses to nursing homes and community care: lessons from Medicaid's history. Georgia State University Law Rev 26(3):937–969

Wilson K (2007) Historical evolution of assisted living in the United States, 1979 to present. Gerontologist 47(1):8–22

Suggested Reading

Rivard C, Rebay K (2012) The 5 mega-trends that are changing the face of health care. Retrieved from https://www.theatlantic.com/health/archive/2012/05/the-5-mega-trends-that-are-changing-the-face-of-health-care/256854/

The Aspen Institute (2012) Reinventing health care. The barriers to innovation. Retrieved from https://assets.aspeninstitute.org/content/uploads/files/content/docs/pubs/hbss-reinventing-hc.pdf

The Eden Alternative (2016) About. Retrieved from http://www.edenalt.org/about-the-eden-alternative/

Licensed Practical Nurse Practice Acts Across the Country

12

12.1   Introduction

This chapter provides information regarding each of the Licensed Practical Nurse Practice Acts in the United States and territories. You also have links to obtain additional information in each state and territory included here.

All states are represented. Only the territories with information regarding the nurse practice act for that territory are included (see Tables 12.1, 12.2, 12.3, 12.4, 12.5, 12.6, 12.7, 12.8, 12.9, 12.10, 12.11, 12.12, 12.13, 12.14, 12.15, 12.16, 12.17, 12.18, 12.19, 12.20, 12.21, 12.22, 12.23, 12.24, 12.25, 12.26, 12.27, 12.28, 12.29, 12.30, 12.31, 12.32, 12.33, 12.34, 12.35, 12.36, 12.37, 12.38, 12.39, 12.40, 12.41, 12.42, 12.43, 12.44, 12.45, 12.46, 12.47, 12.48, 12.49, 12.50, 12.51, 12.52, 12.53).

Table 12.1 Alabama

National Council of State Boards of Nursing (2017). Find your nurse practice act: Alabama. Retrieved from https://www.ncsbn.org/npa.htm
Alabama Board of Nursing (2017). Nurse practice act. Retrieved from http://www.abn.alabama.gov/wp-content/uploads/2016/02/Nursing-Practice-Act-Article-1.pdf
Alabama Nurse Practice Act: Section 34-21-1 Definitions
34-21-1-3b Practice of Practical Nursing
"Practice of Practical Nursing. The performance, for compensation, of acts designed to promote and maintain health, prevent illness and injury and provide care utilizing standardized procedures and the nursing process, including administering medications and treatments, under the direction of a licensed professional nurse or a licensed or otherwise legally authorized physician or dentist. Such practice requires basic knowledge of the biological, physical, and behavioral sciences and of nursing skills but does not require the substantial specialized skill, independent judgment, and knowledge required in the practice of professional nursing. Additional acts requiring appropriate education and training may be performed under emergency or other conditions which are recognized by the nursing and medical professions as proper to be performed by a licensed practical nurse" (Alabama Nurse Practice Act, 2017, p. 1)

© Springer International Publishing AG 2018

C. Kruschke, *Leadership Skills for Licensed Practical Nurses Working with the Aging Population*, https://doi.org/10.1007/978-3-319-69862-5_12

Table 12.2 Alaska

National Council of State Boards of Nursing (2017). Find your nurse practice act: Alaska. Retrieved from https://www.ncsbn.org/npa.htm

Department of Commerce, Community, and Economic Development, Alaska Board of Nursing (2016). Statutes and Regulations Nursing. Retrieved from https://www.commerce.alaska.gov/web/Portals/5/pub/NursingStatutes.pdf

Alaska Nurse Practice Act: Nursing Statutes, AS 08.68

Sec. 08.68.230b. Use of Title and Abbreviation

"A person licensed to practice practical nursing in the state may use the title "licensed practical nurse" and the abbreviation "LPN" (p. 4)

Sec. 08.68.265. Supervision of Practical Nurses

"A practical nurse shall work under the supervision of a licensed registered or advanced practice registered nurse, a licensed physician, a licensed physician assistant, or a licensed dentist" (p. 4)

Sec. 08.68.805. Delegation of Nursing Functions

"A registered, advanced practice registered, or practical nurse licensed under this chapter may delegate nursing duties to other persons, including unlicensed assistive personnel, under regulations adopted by the board. A person to whom the nursing duties are delegated may perform the delegated duties without a license or certificate under this chapter if the person meets the applicable requirements established by the board" (p. 9)

Sec. AS 08.68.850. Definitions

Sec. AS 08.68.850 (8)

"Practice of practical nursing" means the performance for compensation or personal profit of nursing functions that do not require the substantial specialized skill, judgment, and knowledge of a registered nurse (p. 11)

12 AAC 44.990. Definitions

12 AAC 44.990 (18)

"Focused assessment of a patient by a licensed practical nurse means an appraisal of the patient's medical status and condition, contributing to ongoing data collection, and deciding who needs to be informed of the information and when to inform" (p. 9)

Table 12.3 Arizona

National Council of State Boards of Nursing (2017). Find your nurse practice act: Arizona. Retrieved from https://www.ncsbn.org/npa.htm

Arizona State Board of Nursing (2017). Nurse Practice Act. Retrieved from https://www.azbn. gov/laws-rules/nurse-practice-act/

A licensed practical nurse shall engage in practical nursing as defined in A.R.S. 32-1601 only under the supervision of RN or licensed physician. A LPN nursing practice is limited to those activities for which the LPN has been prepared through basic practical nursing education in accordance with A.R.S. 32-1637 (1) and those additional skills that are obtained through subsequent nursing education

A LPN shall:

Contribute to the assessment of the health status of clients to include the following: recognize characteristics that may affect client health status, gather and record assessment data, and demonstrate attentiveness by observing, monitoring, and reporting signs, symptoms, and changes in client condition in ongoing manner that supervising RN or physician

Contribute to the development and modification of plan of care by planning episodic nursing care for client whose condition is stable or predictable, assisting RN or supervising physician in identification of client needs to answer goals, and determining priorities of care together with the supervising RN or physician

Implement aspects of client's care consistent with LPN scope of practice in timely and accurate manner including the following: follow nurse and physician orders and seek clarification of orders when needed; administer treatments, medications, and procedures; attend to client and family concerns or requests; provide health info to clients as directed by supervising RN or physician according to an established educational plan; promote safe client environment; and communicate relevant and timely client info to other health team members regarding client status and progress, client response or lack of response to therapies, significant changes in client condition and client needs, and special requests that contribute to plan of care by gathering, observing, recording, and communicating client responses to nursing interventions and modify plan of care in collaboration with RN based on an analysis of client responses

Table 12.4 Arkansas

National Council of State Boards of Nursing (2017). Find your nurse practice act: Arkansas. Retrieved from https://www.ncsbn.org/npa.htm

Arkansas State Board of Nursing (2015). Nurse practice act of the state of Arkansas. Retrieved from http://www.arsbn.org/Websites/arsbn/images/NursePracticeAct.July.2015.pdf

17-87-102. Definitions

(9) "Practice of licensed practical nursing" means the performance for compensation of nursing practices by a licensed practical nurse that are relevant to the care of the ill, injured, or infirm, or the delegation of certain nursing practices to other personnel as set forth in regulations established by the Board, under the direction of a registered nurse, an advanced practice registered nurse, a licensed physician, or a licensed dentist, that do not require the substantial specialized skill, judgment and knowledge required in professional nursing" (p. 3)

Table 12.5 California

National Council of State Boards of Nursing (2017). Find your nurse practice act: California. Retrieved from https://www.ncsbn.org/npa.htm
California Board of Registered Nursing (2015). California legislative information. Chapter 6.5 Vocational Nursing [2840-2895.5], Article 2. Scope of regulation [2859-2873.6]. Retrieved from http://leginfo.legislature.ca.gov/faces/codes_displayText.xhtml?lawCode=BPC&division= 2.&title=&part=&chapter=6.5.&article=2
Board of Vocational Nursing and Psychiatric Technicians (2015). *Vocational nursing practice act with rules and regulations*. Retrieved from http://www.bvnpt.ca.gov/pdf/vnregs.pdf
2860.5
"A licensed vocational nurse when directed by a physician and surgeon may do all of the following:
(a) Administer medications by hypodermic injection.
(b) Withdraw blood from a patient, if prior thereto such nurse has been instructed by a physician and surgeon and has demonstrated competence to such physician and surgeon in the proper procedure to be employed when withdrawing blood, or has satisfactorily completed a prescribed course of instruction approved by the board, or has demonstrated competence to the satisfaction of the board.
(c) Start and superimpose intravenous fluids if all of the following additional conditions exist:
(1) The nurse has satisfactorily completed a prescribed course of instruction approved by the board or has demonstrated competence to the satisfaction of the board.
(2) The procedure is performed in an organized health care system in accordance with the written standardized procedures adopted by the organized health care system as formulated by a committee which includes representatives of the medical, nursing, and administrative staffs. "Organized health care system," as used in this section, includes facilities licensed pursuant to Section 1250 of the Health and Safety Code, clinics, home health agencies, physician's offices, and public or community health services. Standardized procedures so adopted will be reproduced in writing and made available to total medical and nursing staffs" (Board of Vocational Nursing and Psychiatric Technicians, 2015, p. 5)(*Amended by Stats. 1974, Ch. 1084*)
2860.7
"(a) A licensed vocational nurse, acting under the direction of a physician may perform: (1) tuberculin skin tests, coccidioidin skin tests, and histoplasmin skin tests, providing such administration is within the course of a tuberculosis control program, and (2) immunization techniques, providing such administration is upon standing orders of a supervising physician, or pursuant to written guidelines adopted by a hospital or medical group with whom the supervising physician is associated.
(b) The supervising physician under whose direction the licensed vocational nurse is acting pursuant to subdivision (a) shall require such nurse to:
(1) Satisfactorily demonstrate competence in the administration of immunizing agents, including knowledge of all indications and contraindications for the administration of such agents, and in the recognition and treatment of any emergency reactions to such agents which constitute a danger to the health or life of the person receiving the immunization; and
(2) Possess such medications and equipment as required, in the medical judgment of the supervising physician and surgeon, to treat any emergency conditions and reactions caused by the immunizing agents and which constitute a danger to the health or life of the person receiving the immunization and to demonstrate the ability to administer such medications and to utilize such equipment as necessary.
(c) Nothing in this section shall be construed to require physical presence of a directing or supervising physician, or the examination by a physician of persons to be tested or immunized" (Board of Vocational Nursing and Psychiatric Technicians, 2015, p. 5–6). (*Added by Stats. 1974, Ch. 837*)
2861
"This chapter does not prohibit the performance of nursing services by any person not licensed under this chapter; provided, that such person shall not in any way assume to practice as a licensed vocational nurse" (Board of Vocational Nursing and Psychiatric Technicians, 2015, p. 6). (*Added by Stats. 1951, Ch. 1689*)

Table 12.6 Colorado

National Council of State Boards of Nursing (2017). Find your nurse practice act: Colorado. Retrieved from https://www.ncsbn.org/npa.htm
Colorado Department of Regulatory Agencies (2017). Scope of practice for Licensed Practical Nurses (LPNs). Retrieved from https://www.colorado.gov/pacific/dora/Nursing_Laws
Colorado Department of Regulatory Agencies (2016). Colorado revised statutes, Title 12: Professions and occupations, Article 38: Nurses. Retrieved from file://C:/Users/ckruschk/Downloads/Nurses%20Practice%20Act%20(1).pdf
"The Nurse Practice Act defines the scope of practice of the licensed practical nurse (LPN) as that which is taught in schools of practical nursing in Colorado at this time. Therefore, all decisions regarding tasks that may be performed by a LPN are based on the present curriculum criteria. The LPN curriculum in Colorado is a 9 to 11 month course focusing on the care of patients with predictable outcomes. The curriculum emphasizes the maintenance of those patients and performance of nursing skills with a high degree of technical expertise. The practical nursing student is taught to identify normal from abnormal in each of the body systems and to identify changes in the patient's condition, which are then reported to the RN or MD for further or "full" assessment. For further information regarding the specific tasks and skills taught in the LPN curriculum, you may contact one of the many Colorado colleges offering a LPN program" (Colorado Department of Regulatory Agencies, 2017, para. 4)
Section 12-38-103 (8) Definitions of Practice of Practical Nursing
(8) "Practical nurse," "trained practical nurse," "licensed vocational nurse," or "licensed practical nurse" means a person who holds a license to practice pursuant to the provisions of this article as a licensed practical nurse in this state or is licensed in another state and is practicing in this state pursuant to section 24-60-3202, C.R.S., with the right to use the title "licensed practical nurse" and its abbreviation, "LPN" (Colorado Department of Regulatory Agencies, 2016, p. 2)
Section 12-38-103 (9)(a) Definitions of Practice of Practical Nursing
(9) (a) "Practice of practical nursing" means the performance, under the supervision of a dentist, physician, podiatrist, or professional nurse authorized to practice in this state, of those services requiring the education, training, and experience, as evidenced by knowledge, abilities, and skills required in this article for licensing as a practical nurse pursuant to Section 12-38-112, in (I) caring for the ill, injured, or infirm; (II) teaching and promoting preventive health measures; (III) acting to safeguard life and health; or (IV) administering treatments and medications prescribed by (A) a legally authorized dentist, podiatrist, or physician or (B) physician assistant implementing a medical plan pursuant to subsection (4) of this section. (b) "Practice of practical nursing" includes the performance of delegated medical functions. (c) Nothing in this article shall limit or deny a practical nurse from supervising other practical nurses or other health-care personnel" (Colorado Department of Regulatory Agencies, 2016, p. 3)

Table 12.7 Connecticut

National Council of State Boards of Nursing (2017). Find your nurse practice act: Connecticut. Retrieved from https://www.ncsbn.org/npa.htm
Connecticut Nurses Association (2017). Nurse practice act. Retrieved from http://www.ctnurses.org/Main-Menu-Category/Nursing-Practice/Nurse-Practice-Act/Chapter378Definitions.html#Sec20-87a.htm
Sec. 20-87. Definitions. Section 20-87 is repealed
"(c) The practice of nursing by a licensed practical nurse is defined as the performing of selected tasks and sharing of responsibility under the direction of a registered nurse or an advanced practice registered nurse and within the framework of supportive and restorative care, health counseling and teaching, case finding and referral, collaborating in the implementation of the total health care regimen and executing the medical regimen under the direction of a licensed physician or dentist" (Connecticut Nurses Association, 2017, para. 3)
"(d) In the case of a registered or licensed practical nurse employed by a home health care agency, the practice of nursing includes, but is not limited to, executing the medical regimen under the direction of a physician licensed in a state that borders Connecticut" (Connecticut Nurses Association, 2017, para. 4)

Table 12.8 Delaware

National Council of State Boards of Nursing (2017). Find your nurse practice act: Delaware. Retrieved from https://www.ncsbn.org/npa.htm

Delaware Division of Professional Regulation (2017). 1900 Board of Nursing. Retrieved from http://regulations.delaware.gov/AdminCode/title24/1900.shtml

7.5 Standards of Practice for the Licensed Practical Nurse

7.5.1 "Standards related to the licensed practical nurse's contributions to the nursing process

7.5.1.1 At the direction and under the supervision of a recognized licensed authority, the licensed practical nurse shall contribute to the nursing process and document nursing assessments of individuals and groups by:

7.5.1.1.1 Collecting objective and subjective data from observations, examinations, interview, and written records in an accurate and timely manner. The data include but are not limited to:

7.5.1.1.1.1 Biophysical and emotional status and observed changes

7.5.1.1.1.2 Growth and development

7.5.1.1.1.3 Ethno-cultural, spiritual, socioeconomic, and ecological background

7.5.1.1.1.4 Family health history

7.5.1.1.1.5 Information collected by other health team members

7.5.1.1.1.6 Ability to perform activities of daily living

7.5.1.1.1.7 Consideration of client's health goals

7.5.1.1.1.8 Client knowledge and perception about health status and potential or maintaining health status

7.5.1.1.1.9 Available and accessible human and material resources

7.5.1.1.1.10 Patterns of coping and interaction

7.5.1.1.2 Sorting, selecting, reporting, and recording the data

7.5.1.1.3 Analyzing data

7.5.1.1.4 Validating, refining, and modifying the data by using available resources including interactions with the client, family, significant others, and health team members

7.5.1.2 Licensed practical nurses shall participate in establishing and documenting nursing diagnoses that serve as the basis for the strategy of care

7.5.1.3 Licensed practical nurses shall participate in developing strategies of care based on assessment and nursing diagnoses

7.5.1.3.1 Contributing to setting realistic and measurable goals for implementation

7.5.1.3.2 Participating in identifying measures to maintain comfort, to support human functions and responses to maintain an environment conducive to well-being, and to provide health teaching and counseling

7.5.1.3.3 Contributing to setting client priorities

7.5.1.4 Licensed practical nurses shall participate in the implementation of the strategy of care by:

7.5.1.4.1 Providing care for clients whose conditions are stabilized or predictable

7.5.1.4.2 Providing care for clients whose conditions are critical and/or fluctuating, under the directions and supervision of a recognized licensed authority

7.5.1.4.3 Providing an environment conducive to safety and health

7.5.1.4.4 Documenting nursing interventions and outcomes

7.5.1.4.5 Communicating nursing interventions and outcomes to appropriate health team members

7.5.1.5 Licensed practical nurses shall contribute to evaluating outcomes through appropriate documentation and communication" (Delaware Division of Professional Regulation, 2017, p. 27–28)

Table 12.8 (continued)

7.6.2 Authority to Dispense

7.6.2.2 "Licensed practice nurses may assume the responsibility of dispensing as authorized by the Nurse Practice Act and defined in these regulations, Section 7.6.2.2.1, 7.6.2.2.2, and 7.6.2.2.3

7.6.2.2.1 Licensed practical nurses may provide to a patient prepackaged medications in accordance with the order of a practitioner duly licensed to prescribe medication where such medications have been prepackaged by a person with lawful authority to dispense drugs

7.6.2.2.2 Licensed practical nurses, per written order of a physician, dentist, podiatrist, advanced practice nurse, or other practitioner duly licensed to prescribe medication, may add the name of the client to a preprinted label on a prepackaged medication

7.6.2.2.3 Licensed practical nurses in a licensed methadone clinic may apply a preprinted label to a prepackaged medication" (Delaware Division of Professional Regulation, 2017, p. 28)

7.7.3 Functional Scope of Responsibility for Intravascular Therapy Procedures

7.7.3.4 "The licensed practical nurse is permitted to perform the following procedures for subcutaneous infusions after documented instruction and competency demonstration:

7.7.3.4.1 Accept subcutaneous infusion therapy order(s)

7.7.3.4.2 Insert and remove subcutaneous needle or catheter to initiate/discontinue therapy or rotate sites

7.7.3.4.3 Confirm medication dosage and infusion rate

7.7.3.4.4 Calculate and adjust flow rates on subcutaneous infusion including pumps. This does not include titration nor administration of medications via the "push" route

7.7.3.4.5 Perform dressing and tubing changes

7.7.3.4.6 Maintain subcutaneous infusion therapy

7.7.3.4.7 Change the administration set and convert a continuous infusion to an intermittent infusion and vice versa

7.7.3.4.8 Observe, document, and report on insertion site and signs of complications such as infection, phlebitis, etc." (Delaware Division of Professional Regulation, 2017, p. 30)

7.7.3 Functional Scope of Responsibility for Intravascular Therapy Procedures

7.7.3.2 "Licensed practical nurses bear the responsibility and accountability for their nursing practice under the license granted by the board of Nursing and are permitted to perform the following for peripheral lines:

7.7.3.2.1 Acceptance and confirmation of intravascular therapy order(s)

7.7.3.2.2 Calculation of medication dosage and infusion rate of intravascular medications prescribed. This does not include titration

7.7.3.2.3 Confirmation of medication dosage and infusion rate for intravascular therapy administration

7.7.3.2.4 Add medications in intravascular solutions, label, and document appropriately

7.7.3.2.5 Venipuncture with needle device to establish access to the peripheral vascular system

7.7.3.2.6 Start initial solution or add replacement fluids to an existing infusion as prescribed

7.7.3.2.7 Intravascular therapy maintenance including the flushing of peripheral lines with heparin and/or saline solution

7.7.3.2.8 Termination of peripheral intravascular therapy

7.7.3.2.9 Performance of venipuncture for the purpose of the withdrawal of blood and to monitor the patient's condition before, during, and after the withdrawal of blood"
(Delaware Division of Professional Regulation, 2017, p. 30–31)

(continued)

Table 12.8 (continued)

7.7.3 Functional Scope of Responsibility for Intravascular Therapy Procedures
7.7.3.3 The licensed practical nurse is permitted to perform the following procedures for central lines:
7.7.3.3.1 Acceptance of intravascular therapy order(s)
7.7.3.3.2 Calculation of medication dosage and infusion rate of intravascular medications prescribed. This does not include titration
7.7.3.3.3 Confirmation of medication dosage and infusion rate for intravascular therapy administration
7.7.3.3.4 Add medications in intravascular solutions, label, and document appropriately
7.7.3.3.5 Intravascular therapy maintenance, including the flushing of central lines with heparin and/or saline solution
7.7.3.3.6 Dressing and tubing changes, including PICC lines
7.7.3.3.7 Addition of replacement fluids to an existing infusion as prescribed (Delaware Division of Professional Regulation, 2017, p. 31)

7.7.3 Functional Scope of Responsibility for Intravascular Therapy Procedures
7.7.3.4 The licensed practical nurse is permitted to perform the following procedures for subcutaneous infusions after documented instruction and competency demonstration:
7.7.3.4.1 Accept subcutaneous infusion therapy order(s)
7.7.3.4.2 Insert and remove subcutaneous needle or catheter to initiate/discontinue therapy or rotate sites
7.7.3.4.3 Confirm medication dosage and infusion rate
7.7.3.4.4 Calculate and adjust flow rates on subcutaneous infusion including pumps. This does not include titration nor administration of medications via the "push" route
7.7.3.4.5 Perform dressing and tubing changes
7.7.3.4.6 Maintain subcutaneous infusion therapy
7.7.3.4.7 Change the administration set and convert a continuous infusion to an intermittent infusion and vice versa
7.7.3.4.8 Observe, document, and report on insertion site and signs of complications such as infection, phlebitis, etc. (Delaware Division of Professional Regulation, 2017, p. 31)

Table 12.9 District of Columbia

National Council of State Boards of Nursing (2017). Find your nurse practice act: District of Columbia. Retrieved from https://www.ncsbn.org/npa.htm

DC.gov, Department of Health (2012). Chapter 55: Nursing Licensed Practical Nurses. Retrieved from https://doh.dc.gov/sites/default/files/dc/sites/doh/publication/attachments/Nursing_Licensed_Practical_Nurses.pdf

5514 Scope of Practice

5514.1 The practice of practical nursing means the following:

(a) "The performance of actions of preventive health care, health maintenance, and the care of persons who are ill, injured, or experiencing alterations in health processes at the direction of the delegating or supervisory registered nurse

(b) The basic knowledge, judgment, and skills in nursing procedures gained through successful completion of an approved educational program in practical nursing" (DC.gov, Department of Health, 2012, p. 16)

5514 Scope of Practice

5514.2 A practical nurse shall accept only those assigned nursing activities and responsibilities as set forth in the act and this chapter, which the practical nurse can safely perform. That acceptance shall be based on the following requirements in each practice setting which shall include:

(a) "The qualifications of the practical nurse in relation to the client's needs and the integrated plan of care, including:

(1) Basic education and preparation of the practical nurse

(2) Knowledge and skills subsequently acquired through continuing education and practice

(b) The degree of supervision by a registered nurse

(c) The stability of each of the clients' condition

(d) The complexity and frequency of nursing intervention to address the needs of the client or client group

(e) The accessible resources within the agency or facility

(f) The established policies, procedures, standards of practice, and communication channels, which lend support to the model of nursing services offered by the agency or facility" (DC. gov, Department of Health, 2012, p. 16)

(continued)

Table 12.9 (continued)

5514 Scope of Practice

5514.3 The practice of practical nursing shall include the following:

(a) "Participating in the performance of the ongoing comprehensive nursing assessment process of the client's biological, physiological, and behavioral health, including the client's reaction to an illness, injury, and treatment regimens by collecting data and performing focused nursing assessments

(b) Recording and reporting the findings and results of the ongoing nursing assessment process

(c) Participating in the development and modification of the client-centered plan of care

(d) The administration of medication and treatment as prescribed by a legally authorized health-care professional, licensed in the District of Columbia, and that is within the scope of practice of a practical nurse

(e) Implementing appropriate aspects of the integrated plan of care in which the practical nurse is knowledgeable, skilled, and competent to perform and that is within the scope of practice of the practical nurse

(f) Participating in the nursing care management through assigning and directing nursing interventions that may be performed by unlicensed, trained personnel

(g) Participating in the evaluation of the client response and outcome to interventions

(h) Promoting and maintaining a safe and therapeutic environment

(i) Participating in health teaching and counseling to promote, attain, and maintain the optimum health level of the client

(j) Communicating and collaborating with other health-care team members and other professionals

(k) Monitoring intravenous infusion

(l) Inserting nasogastric tubes

(m) Other acts or services which are beyond the basic education of a practical nurse as approved by the board. The acts or services shall be commensurate with the practical nurse's experience, continuing education, and demonstrated competencies" (DC.gov, Department of Health, 2012, p. 17)

5514 Scope of Practice

5514.5 A practical nurse may administer medications intravenously if the following conditions are met:

(a) "The administrator for nursing services has developed policies, procedures, and practice standards governing the practice of medication administration by practical nurses and established specific criteria for use when approving medications for intravenous administration by practical nurses

(b) The practical nurse has successfully completed an educational program for intravenous medication administration

(c) The practical nurse has been evaluated and validated for clinical competency in intravenous medication administration

(d) The practical nurse administers the approved medications under the general supervision of a licensed, registered nurse" (DC.gov, Department of Health, 2012, p. 18)

5514 Scope of Practice

5514.7 A practical nurse shall only administer medications which have been approved by the administrator for nursing services (DC.gov, Department of Health, 2012, p. 19)

5514 Scope of Practice

5514.8 A practical nurse may perform infusion therapy upon successfully completing an approved program of infusion therapy approved by the board and if the following requirements are met:

(a) "The administrator of nursing services has developed policies, procedures, and practice standards which govern the practice of infusion therapy

(b) The supervisor maintains documentation to validate the competency of the practical nurse

(c) A registered nurse is present in the facility or on the unit when the practical nurse is performing infusion therapy" (DC.gov, Department of Health, 2012, p. 19)

Table 12.9 (continued)

5514 Scope of Practice
5514.9 A practical nurse may perform the following infusion therapy acts:
(a) "Insertion of a peripheral intravenous catheter that is no more than 3 inches in length
(b) Discontinuing peripheral intravenous catheters that are no more than 3 inches in length
(c) Initiation of prescribed intravenous fluids
(d) Calculating and adjusting intravenous flow rate, including infusion pumps
(e) Adding intravenous fluids to an established peripheral line. Fluids must be nonmedicated, commercially prepared, or prepared by a licensed pharmacist. Accepted fluids are limited to those fluids that are generally used as maintenance and isotonic in nature
(f) Administering pharmacy-prepared medications
(g) Insertion of heparin locks, including flushing with normal saline or heparin 100 units
(h) Venipuncture or withdrawal of a blood specimen from a peripheral catheter site
(i) Changing of injection cap or intravenous tubing for peripheral lines only" (DC.gov, Department of Health, 2012, p. 19)

Table 12.10 Florida

National Council of State Boards of Nursing (2017). Find your nurse practice act: Florida. Retrieved from https://www.ncsbn.org/npa.htm
Florida Department of Health (2007). Florida Board of Nursing. Chapter 464 Florida Statutes. Rules of the Board of Nursing. Chapter 64B9 Florida Administrative Code. Retrieved from https://phsc.edu/sites/default/files/program/files/Nurse-Practice-Act.pdf
64B9-12 Florida Administrative Code
64B9-12.001 Statement of Intent and Purpose
464.003 Definitions
Practice of practical nursing performance selected acts including administration of treatments and medications in care of ill, injured, or infirm and promotion of wellness maintenance of health and prevention of illness of others under the direction of RN or licensed physician, osteopathic, podiatric physicians, or licensed dentist
Professional nurse and practical nurse shall be responsible and accountable for making decisions that are based upon individual's preparation and experience in nursing
Chapter 64B9-12 Administration of Intravenous Therapy by Licensed Practical Nurses
64B9-12.001 Statement of Intent and Purpose
(1) "The "practice of practical nursing" as defined by Section 464.003(3)(b), Florida Statutes, includes the "administration of treatments and medication," under direction, and holds the licensed practical nurse "responsible and accountable for making decisions . . . based upon the individual's educational preparation and experience in nursing." As medical science advances and the demands for health care in Florida grow, the scope of nursing practice, in general, and of the practice of practical nursing, in particular, is expanding. It has become necessary that the licensed practical nurse, when qualified by training and education and when approved by the institution at which the licensed practical nurse is employed, engages in the limited administration of intravenous therapy both to serve the public and to allow the professional nurse to better perform those acts requiring professional nursing specialized knowledge, judgment, and skill
(2) The purpose of this rule is to protect the public by ensuring the availability of intravenous therapy and its competent administration in the care of the ill, injured, or the infirm. In keeping with the purpose, this rule authorizes the qualified licensed practical nurse to administer those aspects of intravenous therapy within the scope of practice of the licensed practical nurse, enumerates those aspects of intravenous therapy outside the scope of practice of the licensed practical nurse, and sets out the educational and/or competency verification necessary to administer, under direction, limited forms of intravenous therapy
Specific Authority 464.006 FS. Law Implemented 464.003(3)(b) FS. History–New 1-16-91, Formerly 21O-21.001, 61F7-12.001, 59S-12.001" (Florida Department of Health, 2007, p. 93)

(continued)

Table 12.10 (continued)

64B9-12.004 Authority LPN Administers Limited Forms IV to Include
- Perform calculations and adjust flow
- Observe and report subjective and objective signs of adverse reactions to IV administration
- Inspect insertion site, change dressing, and remove IV needle or catheter from peripheral veins
- Hang bags or bottles of hydrating fluid (Florida Department of Health, 2007, p. 94)

Table 12.11 Georgia

National Council of State Boards of Nursing (2017). Find your nurse practice act: Georgia. Retrieved from https://www.ncsbn.org/npa.htm

State of Georgia (2017). Title 43. Professions and Businesses. Chapter 26: Nurses. Article 1: Georgia registered professional nurse practice act. Article 2: Licensed Practical Nurses, page 18–27. Retrieved from http://sos.ga.gov/PLB/acrobat/Forms/38%20Reference%20-%20Nurse%20Practice%20Act.pdf

Title 43 Professions and Businesses

Chapter 26 Nurse

Article 2: Licensed Practical Nurses

Section 43-26-30

This article shall be known and cited as the "Georgia Practical Nurses Practice Act" (State of Georgia, 2017, p. 18)

Section 43-26-4

(7) "The practice of licensed practical nursing" means provisions of care for compensation, under the supervision of physician practicing medicine, dentist, podiatrist, or RN in accordance to applicable provisions of law. Relates to maintenance of health and prevention of illness shall include but are not limited to:

A. Participate in assessment, planning, implementation, and evaluation of delivery health-care services and other specialized tasks when appropriately trained and consistent with board rules and regulations

B. Provide direct personal patient observation, care, and assistance in hospital, clinics, nursing homes, emergency treatment facilities, or other health-care facility types of care: coronary care, intensive care, emergency treatment, surgical care, recovery, obstetrics, pediatrics, outpatient services, home health care, or other areas of practice such as C, D, and E

C. Perform comfort and safety measures

D. Administer treatments and medications

E. Participate in the management and supervision of unlicensed personnel in the delivery of patient care" (State of Georgia, 2017, p. 20)

Table 12.12 Guam

National Council of State Boards of Nursing (2017). Find your nurse practice act: Guam. Retrieved from https://www.ncsbn.org/npa.htm

10 GCA Health And Safety (2017). Chapter 12: Medical Practices. Retrieved from https://www.ncsbn.org/Guam_npa.pdf

§ 12314. Qualifications for Practical Nurses

a) "An applicant for a license to practice as a licensed practical nurse shall submit to the board a written, verified evidence that the applicant:

   1) Is a graduate of an approved practical nursing program
   2) Has successfully completed courses of study in an approved professional nursing education program, including experience in medical, surgical, obstetrics, and pediatric nursing
   3) Has served on active duty in the military corps of any of the armed forces, in which no less than an aggregate of 12 months was spent in rendering patient care, and who has completed the basic course of instruction in the hospital corps school required by his particular branch of the armed forces, and whose service in the armed forces has been under honorable conditions. This person may submit the record of such training to the board for evaluation

b) If a person meets the necessary qualifications of this Section, he shall be granted a license upon passing the standardized examination for such a licensure. The qualifications are:

   1) That he has completed such general preliminary education requirements as shall be determined by the board
   2) That he has committed no act, which, if committed by a licensee, would be grounds for disciplinary action
   3) That his education and experience would give reasonable assurance of competence to practice as a licensed practical nurse in Guam
   4) The board shall, by regulation, establish criteria for evaluating the education and experience for applicants under this section" (10 GCA Health And Safety, 2017, p. 11–12)

Table 12.13 Hawaii

National Council of State Boards of Nursing (2017). Find your nurse practice act: Hawaii. Retrieved from https://www.ncsbn.org/npa.htm

Department of Commerce and Consumer Affairs. Professional and Vocational Licensing (2017). Chapter 47: Nurses. Retrieved from https://cca.hawaii.gov/pvl/files/2013/08/HRS_457-Nurses0716.pdf

§457-2.6 Licensed Practical Nurse

"Practice as a licensed practical nurse means the directed scope of nursing practice, regardless of compensation or personal profit, that takes place under the direction of a registered nurse, advanced practice registered nurse, licensed physician, or other health-care provider authorized by the state, and is guided by the scope of practice authorized by this chapter, the rules of the board, and nursing standards established or recognized by the board including but not limited to:

(1) The National Council of State Boards of Nursing Model Nursing Practice Act, Article II, Scope of Nursing Practice, Section 3

(2) The National Council of State Boards of Nursing Model Nursing Administrative Rules, Chapter Two, Standards of Nursing Practice, Sections 2.3.1 through 2.3.3, provided the NCSBN, shall have no legal authority over the board and shall have no legal authority or powers of oversight of the board in the exercise of its powers and duties authorized by law" (Department of Commerce and Consumer Affairs. Professional and Vocational Licensing, 2017, p. 4)

Table 12.14 Idaho

National Council of State Boards of Nursing (2017). Find your nurse practice act: Idaho. Retrieved from https://www.ncsbn.org/npa.htm

State of Idaho, Board of Nursing (2017). Rules of the Idaho State Board of Nursing. Retrieved from https://adminrules.idaho.gov/rules/2000/23/0101.pdf

23.01.01 Rules of the Idaho State Board of Nursing

401. Licensed Practical Nurse

"The licensed practical nurse provides nursing care at the direction of a licensed professional nurse, licensed physician, or licensed dentist and under guidelines established by the Board of Nursing and the employing agency. The stability of the environment and clinical state of the client determine the degree of direction and direct supervision that must be provided to the licensed practical nurse. The licensed practical nurse shall be personally accountable and responsible for all actions taken in carrying out nursing activities. The interpretation of functions as set forth in the legal definition of licensed practical nurse, Section 54-1402 (b),(2), Idaho Code, (Nursing Practice Act) is as follows:" (State of Idaho, Board of Nursing, 2017, p. 39)

01. Contributing to the assessment of health status. "The licensed practical nurse contributes to the assessment of health status by collecting, reporting, and recording objective and subjective data. Data collection includes:

   a. Obtaining a health history

   b. Making systematic observations to identify deviations from normal

   c. Identifying signs and symptoms of change in behavior or condition

   d. Identifying need for immediate nursing intervention based upon data collected" (State of Idaho, Board of Nursing, 2017, p. 39)

02. Participating in the development and modification of care. "The licensed practical nurse participates in the development and modification of the strategy of care by:

   a. Recognizing, understanding, and respecting the client's cultural background, spiritual needs, values and beliefs, and right of choice

   b. Identifying common, recurrent health problems (7-1-91)

   c. Identifying priority needs

   d. Identifying major short- and long-term goals or outcomes

   e. Identifying measures to maintain hygiene and comfort, to support human functions, to maintain an environment conducive to safety and well-being, and to provide health instruction

   f. Utilizing data collected to assist in the development of the plan of nursing care" (State of Idaho, Board of Nursing, 2017, p. 39)

Table 12.14 (continued)

03. Implementing aspects of the strategy of care

"The licensed practical nurse implements aspects of the strategy of care by:

  a. Providing direct physical care and comfort measures and emotional support for clients whose conditions are stabilized or predictable

  b. Providing care under the direct supervision of the licensed professional nurse, licensed physician, or licensed dentist, for clients whose conditions are complex or unstable

  c. Assisting the client in activities of daily living and assisting the client in assuming responsibility for self-care

  d. Assisting with the rehabilitation of clients through knowledge and application of principles of supportive therapy and of prevention of deformities, such as the normal range of motion exercises, body mechanics, and body alignment

  e. Providing an environment conducive to safety and health

  f. Assisting with client teaching

  g. Administering prescribed medications through a variety of routes (except by intravenous push), including but not limited to allergy injections and continuous subcutaneous administration of narcotics after client stabilization

  h. Providing prescribed treatments and procedures as are taught in Board-approved curriculum for practical nurses, including but not limited to:

   I. Inserting, monitoring, and caring for various lines and tubes including but not limited to gavage feeding (including infants), nasogastric tubes, and reinsertion of gastrostomy and suprapubic catheters with established tracts and nasotracheal or tracheal tube suctioning

   II. Removing drains and packing, sutures/clips/staples, casts, and Gomco clamps in circumcisions

   III. Performing a variety of procedures including but not limited to application of monitoring equipment, recording of readings, and hemodialysis or peritoneal dialysis

  a. Monitoring responses to medication, intravenous therapy, and treatments

  b. Performing peripheral intravenous therapy functions as follows:

   I. Observing, monitoring, reporting and documenting the status of intravenous sites, and taking appropriate action to minimize or prevent intravenous complications

   II. Hanging containers of medicated or unmedicated intravenous solutions which are commercially prepared or premixed by pharmacy, hanging blood or blood derivatives, inserting analgesic cartridges, programming and monitoring patient-controlled analgesia pumps, and performing autoinfusion

   III. Calculating and maintaining flow rates, adjusting the drip rates on intravenous infusions and pumps, filling solusets and volume controls, changing intravenous tubing, converting an intravenous infusion to a heparin/saline lock, flushing lines, and setting up and managing syringe pump infusions

   IV. Performing vein punctures to draw blood

   V. Discontinuing intravenous infusions

  a. Documenting nursing interventions and responses to care

  b. Communicating nursing interventions and responses to care to appropriate members of the health team

  c. Executing the legal orders of a health-care provider authorized to prescribe medications based on requisite knowledge of the cause and effect of the order. This includes verifying that the order is accurate and that there are no documented contraindications to carrying out the order

  d. Carrying out those duties that may be performed by unlicensed assistive personnel" (State of Idaho, Board of Nursing, 2017, p. 39–40)

Table 12.15 Illinois

National Council of State Boards of Nursing (2017). Find your nurse practice act: Illinois. Retrieved from https://www.ncsbn.org/npa.htm

Illinois General Assembly (2007). Illinois Compiled Statutes. Professions, Occupations, and Business Operations, (225 ILCS 65) Nurse Practice Act. Article 55, Nursing Licensure, Licensed Practical Nurses. Retrieved from http://ilga.gov/legislation/ilcs/ilcs4.asp?DocName=0 22500650HArt%2E+55&ActID=1312&ChapterID=24&SeqStart=14800000&Seq End=15600000

Article 55 Nursing

(225 ILCS 65/55-30) (section scheduled to be repealed on January 1, 2018)

Section 55-30 LPN Scope of Practice

(a) "Practice as a LPN means a scope of basic nursing practice as delegated by a RN or an advanced practice nurse or as directed by PA, physician, dentist, or podiatric physician and includes but is not limited to:

   (1) Collecting data and collaborating in the assessment of health status of patient

   (2) Collaborating in development and modification of the registered professional nurse or advance practice nurse comprehensive nursing plan of care for all types of patients

   (3) Implementing aspects of plan of care as delegated

   (4) Participating in health teaching and counseling to promote, attain, and maintain the health level of patients as delegated

   (5) Service as an advocate for patient by communicating and collaborating with other health service personnel as delegated

   (6) Participating in the evaluation of patient responses to interventions

   (7) Communicating and collaborating with other health-care professionals as delegated

   (8) Provide input into development of policies and procedures to support patient safety" (Illinois General Assembly, 2007, section 6)

Table 12.16 Indiana

National Council of State Boards of Nursing (2017). Find your nurse practice act: Indiana. Retrieved from https://www.ncsbn.org/npa.htm

Indiana General Assembly (2015). IC 25-23: Article 23 Nurses. Retrieved from http://iga. in.gov/legislative/laws/2015/ic/titles/025/articles/023/

Article 23 Nurses

IC 25-23-1-1.2 Licensed Practical Nurse

"Sec. 1.2. As used in this chapter, "licensed practical nurse" means a person who holds a valid license issued under this chapter or by a party state (as defined in IC 25-23.3-2-11) and who functions at the direction of:

   1) A registered nurse

   2) A physician with an unlimited license to practice medicine or osteopathic medicine

   3) A licensed dentist

   4) A licensed chiropractor

   5) A licensed optometrist

   6) A licensed podiatrist

in the performance of activities commonly performed by practical nurses and requiring special knowledge or skill" (Indiana General Assembly, 2015, p. 3–4)

IC 25-23-1-1.3 "Practical Nursing" Defined

"Sec. 1.3. As used in this chapter, "practical nursing" means the performance of services commonly performed by practical nurses, including:

   1) Contributing to the assessment of the health status of individuals or groups

   2) Participating in the development and modification of the strategy of care

   3) Implementing the appropriate aspects of the strategy of care

   4) Maintaining safe and effective nursing care

   5) Participating in the evaluation of responses to the strategy of care" (Indiana General Assembly, 2015, p. 4)

Table 12.17 Iowa

National Council of State Boards of Nursing (2017). Find your nurse practice act: Iowa. Retrieved from https://www.ncsbn.org/npa.htm

Iowa Board of Nursing (2011). Chapter 6 Nursing Practice For Registered Nurses/Licensed Practical Nurses. Retrieved from https://www.legis.iowa.gov/docs/iac/rule/01-12-2011.655.6.3.pdf

Chapter 6 Nursing Practice for RN/LPN

655-6.3 (152) Minimum Standards of Practice for LPN

6.3 (1) "Must understand legal implications within scope of nursing practice. LPN shall perform services in provision of supportive or restorative care under the supervision of RN or physician as defined in Iowa codes" (Iowa Board of Nursing, 2011, p. 3)

6.3 (2)· "LPN shall participate in nursing process consistent with accepted practice by assisting a RN or physician. LPN may assist RN in monitoring, observing, and reporting reactions to therapy" (Iowa Board of Nursing, 2011, p. 3)

6.3 (3): "LPN shall not perform activity requiring knowledge and skills ascribed to RN
  a) Assess related to procedures/therapies requiring knowledge or skill level of RN
  b) Initiation of IV solutions, IV medications, or blood components
  c) Administration of medications requiring knowledge or skill ascribed to RN
  d) Initiation or administration of medications requiring knowledge and skills of RN" (Iowa
     Board of Nursing, 2011, p. 3)

6.3 (4) "LPN under the supervision of RN may engage in limited scope of practice of IV therapy. Limited scope of IV therapy may include:
  a) Addition of IV solutions without adding medications to establish peripheral IV sites
  b) Regulation of rate of nonmedicated IV solutions to establish peripheral IV sites
  c) Administration of maintenance doses of analgesics via the patient-controlled analgesic
     pump at lockout interval to establish peripheral IV sites
  d) Discontinue of peripheral IV therapy
  e) Administration of prefilled heparin or saline syringe flush, prepackaged by the
     manufacturer of premixed and labeled by a registered pharmacist or RN to an established
     peripheral lock, in licensed hospital, nursing facility, or a certified end-stage renal dialysis
     unit" (Iowa Board of Nursing, 2011, p. 3)

6.3 (5) "When nursing tasks are delegated by RN to LPN in certified end-stage renal dialysis unit, the facility must have a written policy that defines the practice and written verification of education and competency of LPN per facility written policy. Nursing tasks which may be delegated to LPN for the sole purpose of hemodialysis treatment include:
  a) Initiation and discontinuation of the hemodialysis treatment using any of the following
     established vascular accesses: central line, arteriovenous fistula, and graft
  b) Administration during hemodialysis treatment of local anesthetic prior to cannulation of
     the vascular site
  c) Administration of prescribed dosages of heparin solution utilized in the initiation and
     discontinuation of hemodialysis
  d) Administration, during hemodialysis treatment via the extra ordeal circuit, of the routine IV
     medication erythropoietin, vitamin D analog, intravenous antibiotic solutions prepackaged by
     the manufacturer or premixed and labeled by registered pharmacist or RN, and iron excluding
     any iron preparation that requires a test dose. The RN shall administer the first dose of
     erythropoietin, vitamin D analog, antibiotics, and iron" (Iowa Board of Nursing, 2011, p. 3)

6.3 (6) "The LPN may provide nursing care in acute care setting. When nursing care provided by LPN in an acute care setting requires knowledge and skill level ascribed to RN, a RN or physician must be present in the proximate area. Acute care settings requiring the knowledge and skills ascribed to RN include but are not limited to:
  a) Units where care of unstable, critically ill, or critically injured patient is provided
  b) General medical surgical units
  c) Emergency departments
  d) Operating rooms (LPN may assist with circulating duties when supervised by RN
     circulating in same room)

(continued)

Table 12.17 (continued)

  e) Postanesthesia recovery units
  f) Hemodialysis units
  g) Labor and delivery/birthing units
  h) Mental health units" (Iowa Board of Nursing, 2011, p. 4)
6.3 (7) "LPN may provide nursing care in a nonacademic care setting. When nursing care
provided by LPN in a non-acute care setting requires knowledge or skill ascribed to RN, the
RN or physician must be present in proximate area. The non-acute care settings requiring
knowledge and skills level ascribed to RN include but are not limited to:
  a) Community health
  b) School nursing
  c) Occupational nursing
  d) Correctional facilities
  e) Community mental health nursing" (Iowa Board of Nursing, 2011, p. 4)
6.3 (8) "The LPN shall conduct nursing practice by respecting rights of individual or group"
(Iowa Board of Nursing, 2011, p. 4)
6.3 (9) "LPN shall conduct nursing practice by respecting confidentiality of an individual or
group, unless obligated to disclose proper authorization or legal compulsion" (Iowa Board of
Nursing, 2011, p. 4)
6.3 (10) "LPN shall recognize and understand the legal implications of accountability.
Accountability includes but is not limited to:
  a) Perform activities and functions requiring knowledge and skills currently ascribed to LPN
     and seeking assistance when activities and functions are beyond licensees scope of
     preparation
  b) Accept responsibility for performing assigned and delegated functions and informing the
     RN when assigned and delegated functions are not executed
  c) Executing medical regime prescribed by physician. In executing said regime, LPN shall
     exercise prudent judgment in accordance with minimum standards of nursing practice
     defined in these rules. If medical regime is not carried out based on LPN's prudent
     judgment, accountability shall include but not limited to:
     1) Timely notification of physician who prescribed medical regime that said order was not
        executed and reasons for same
     2) Documentation on medical record that physician was notified and reasons for not
        executing orders
  d) Wear identification identifying LPN when providing direct patient care" (Iowa Board of
     Nursing, 2011, p. 4)
655-6.5(152) Additional Acts Performed by LPN
"LPN shall supervise unlicensed assisting personnel that includes any or all of the following:
direct observation of a function or activity, delegation of nursing tasks while retaining
accountability, and determination that nursing care being provided is adequate and delivered
appropriately
  a) Supervision shall be in accordance with:
     1) LPN working under the supervision of RN is permitted to supervise an intermediate
        care facility for mentally retarded or in residential health-care setting
     2) LPN under the supervision of RN shall be permitted to supervise in nursing facility. The
        LPN shall be required to complete curriculum approved by board designed for
        supervision role
     3) LPN can supervise without educational requirement if LPN was performing supervisory
        role on or before October 6, 1982. LPN employed in supervisory role after the enactment
        of rules shall complete the curriculum" (Iowa Board of Nursing, 2011, p. 5)
     4) LPN working under the supervision of RN may direct activities of other LPN and
        unlicensed assistive personnel in an acute care setting giving care to individuals
        assigned to LPN. RN must be in the proximate area"
6.5(2) "LPN can practice as diagnostic radiographer while under the supervision of a licensed
practitioner provided that training standards for use of radiation-emitting equipment are met"
(Iowa Board of Nursing, 2011, p. 6)

Table 12.17   (continued)

6.5(3) "LPN is permitted to perform in addition to 6.3 (4) procedures related to expanded scope of practice of IV therapy upon completion of board-approved expanded IV therapy certification course" (Iowa Board of Nursing, 2011, p. 6)

655-6.6 (152) Specific Nursing Practice for LPN
6.6(1) "LPN permitted to provide supportive and restorative care in home setting under the supervision of RN or physician; initial assessment and ongoing application shall be provided by RN
6.6(2) LPN can provide supportive and restorative care in school setting, head start program, camp setting, and county jail all under the supervision of RN or physician. RN to perform initial assessments, etc." (Iowa Board of Nursing, 2011, p. 7)

Table 12.18   Kansas

National Council of State Boards of Nursing (2017). Find your nurse practice act: Kansas. Retrieved from https://www.ncsbn.org/npa.htm

Kansas State Board of Nursing (2016). Nurse practice act. Statutes and administrative regulations. Retrieved from http://www.ksbn.org/npa/npa.pdf

65-1113 Definitions (d) Practice of Nursing
(2) "The practice of nursing as LPN means performance for compensation or gratuitously except as permitted by KSA 65-1124 and any amendments of tasks and responsibilities defined in part (1) of this subsection (d) which tasks and responsibilities are based on acceptable educational preparation within framework of supportive and restorative care under the direction of RN, a person licensed to practice medicine and surgery, or a person licensed to practice dentistry" (Kansas State Board of Nursing, 2016, p. 12)

60-16-102. Scope of Practice for Licensed Practical Nurse Performing Intravenous Fluid Therapy
a) "A licensed practical nurse under the supervision of a registered professional nurse may engage in a limited scope of intravenous fluid treatment, including the following:
   1) Monitoring
   2) Maintaining basic fluids
   3) Discontinuing intravenous flow and an intravenous access device not exceeding 3 inches in length in peripheral sites only
   4) Changing dressings for intravenous access devices not exceeding 3 inches in length in peripheral sites only" (Kansas State Board of Nursing, 2016, p. 44)

Table 12.19   Kentucky

National Council of State Boards of Nursing (2017). Find your nurse practice act: Kentucky. Retrieved from https://www.ncsbn.org/npa.htm

Kentucky Board of Nursing (2017). RN/LPN scope of practice determination guidelines. Retrieved from https://kbn.ky.gov/practice/Documents/ScopeDeterminGuidelines.pdf

KRS Chapter 314
KRS 314.011(10) "defines LPN practice as performance of acts required. Knowledge and skill as taught or acquired in approved schools include:
   a) Observe and care for ill, injured, or infirmed under the direction of RN, advanced practice RN, PA, licensed physician, or dentist
   b) Give counsel and apply procedures to safeguard life and health as defined by authorized board
   c) Administer medications and treatments as authorized by physicians, PA, dentist, or advanced practice RN and further authorized or limited by the board which is consistent NY nationally accepted organizations of LPN
   d) Teach, supervise, and delegate except as limited by the board
   e) Perform other nursing acts consistent with the National Federation of LPN standards of practice established by nationally accepted organization of LPN" (Kentucky Board of Nursing, 2017, p. 1)

Table 12.20 Louisiana

National Council of State Boards of Nursing (2017). Find your nurse practice act: Louisiana. Retrieved from https://www.ncsbn.org/npa.htm

Louisiana State Legislature (2017). Part II. Practical Nurses. Retrieved from https://legis.la.gov/Legis/Law.aspx?d=94527

Part II. Part II. Practical Nurses

§961. §961. Definitions

"As used in this part:

(1) "Accredited school" means a school of practical nursing approved by the board

(2) "Board" means the Louisiana State Board of Practical Nurse Examiners

(3) "Practical nurse" means a person who practices practical nursing and who is licensed to practice under this part

(4) The "practice of practical nursing" means the performance for compensation of any acts, not requiring the education, training, and preparation required in professional nursing, in the care, treatment, or observation of persons who are ill, injured, or infirm and for the maintenance of the health of others and the promotion of health care, including the administration of medications and treatments or in on-the-job training or supervising licensed practical nurses, subordinate personnel, or instructing patients consistent with the licensed practical nurse's education and preparation, under the direction of a licensed physician, optometrist, dentist acting individually or in his capacity as a member of the medical staff, or registered nurse. The licensed practical nurse may perform any of the foregoing duties and with appropriate training may perform additional specified acts which are authorized by the Louisiana State Board of Practical Nurse Examiners when directed to do so by the licensed physician, optometrist, dentist acting individually or in his capacity as a member of the medical staff, or registered nurse" (Louisiana State Legislature, 2017, para. 1)

Table 12.21 Maine

National Council of State Boards of Nursing (2017). Find your nurse practice act: Maine. Retrieved from https://www.ncsbn.org/npa.htm

Maine Legislature (2017). Title 32, Chapter 31: Nurses and Nursing. Retrieved from http://legislature.maine.gov/legis/statutes/32/title32ch31sec0.html

Title 32: Professions and Occupations

Chapter 31: Nurses and Nursing

Subchapter 1: General Provisions

§2102 Definitions

3. Practical nursing. "The practice of 'practical nursing' means performing tasks and responsibilities, by a licensed practical nurse, for compensation within a structured health care setting, reinforcing the patient and family teaching program through health teaching, health counseling and provision of supportive and restorative care, under the direction of a registered nurse or licensed or otherwise legally authorized physician, podiatrist or dentist" (Maine Legislature, 2017, para. 22)

Table 12.22 Maryland

National Council of State Boards of Nursing (2017). Find your nurse practice act: Maryland. Retrieved from https://www.ncsbn.org/npa.htm

Thomas Reuter's Westlaw (2015). West's annotated code of Maryland health occupations. Retrieved from https://govt.westlaw.com/mdc/Document/N34F7E791303511E58C09C6D9E4B 64EFE?viewType=FullText&originationContext=documenttoc&transitionType=CategoryPageI tem&contextData=(sc.Default)

Practice Licensed Practical Nursing

(m) "Practice licensed practical nursing means to perform in a team relationship an act that requires specialized knowledge, judgment, and skill based on principles of biological, physiological, behavioral, or sociological science to:

(1) Administer treatment or medication to an individual;

(2) Aid in the rehabilitation of an individual;

(3) Promote preventive measures in community health;

(4) Give counsel to an individual;

(5) Safeguard life and health;

(6) Teach or supervise; or

(7) Perform any additional acts authorized by the Board under § 8-205 of this title" (Thomas Reuter's Westlaw, 2015, para. 13)

Table 12.23 Massachusetts

National Council of State Boards of Nursing (2017). Find your nurse practice act: Massachusetts. Retrieved from https://www.ncsbn.org/npa.htm

The 190th General Court of the Commonwealth of Massachusetts (2017). Section 80B: Nursing practice; advanced practice; licensed practical nurses. Retrieved from https:// malegislature.gov/Laws/GeneralLaws/PartI/TitleXVI/Chapter112/Section80B

Section 80B Nursing Practice, Advanced Practice, and Licensed Practical Nurses

"The practice of LPN shall include but is not limited to:

1) Participation in the development, implementation, evaluation, and modification of the plans of nursing care for individuals, families, and communities through the application of nursing theory;

2) Participation in the coordination and management of resources for the delivery of patient care;

3) Managing, directing, and supervising safe and effective nursing care, including the delegation of selective activities to unlicensed assisting personnel (The 190th General Court of the Commonwealth of Massachusetts, 2017, para. 10).

Neither "professional nursing" nor "practical nursing" shall mean or be construed to prevent

1) The gratuitous care of any ill, injured, or infirm person by any member of his family or any friend or his care by any person employed primarily as a companion, housekeeper, domestic servant, or nurse maid

2) The performance of any nursing service in an emergency

3) The performance of any student enrolled in a school for nurses or practical nurses duly approved in accordance with this chapter, of any nursing service to any prescribed course in such school

4) The performance of services incidental to the Practice of the religious tenets of any church by any member thereof

5) The performance of nursing service by a person authorized to practice under section 76A, subject the provisions of said section or

6) The performance of services by physicians, dentists, pharmacists, teachers, health educators, social workers, dieticians, therapists, technicians, and medical students which are commonly recognized Tobe functions of their respective callings

7) Through performance of any nursing service for any patient in a convalescent or nursing home or rest home, by any person employed in such home, provided that such nursing service is performed under the supervision of an RN or licensed practical nurse" (The 190th General Court of the Commonwealth of Massachusetts, 2017, para. 11)

Table 12.24 Michigan

National Council of State Boards of Nursing (2017). Find your nurse practice act: Michigan. Retrieved from https://www.ncsbn.org/npa.htm

Department of Licensing and Regulatory Affairs (1978). Public health code, Act 368 of 1978. Retrieved from http://www.legislature.mi.gov/documents/mcl/pdf/mcl-act-368-of-1978.pdf

Public Health Code
Act 368 of 1978
Part 172 Nursing
333.17201: Definitions and Principles of Construction
Sec 17201 (1)(d)
(d) "Practice of nursing as a 'licensed practical nurse' or 'l.p.n.' means the practice of nursing based on less comprehensive knowledge and skill than that required of a registered professional nurse and performed under the supervision of a registered professional nurse, physician, or dentist" (Department of Licensing and Regulatory Affairs, 1978, p. 416)

Table 12.25 Minnesota

National Council of State Boards of Nursing (2017). Find your nurse practice act: Minnesota. Retrieved from https://www.ncsbn.org/npa.htm

Minnesota Board of Nursing (2013). Nurse practice act. Minnesota statue section 148.171. Retrieved from https://mn.gov/boards/assets/NPA_2013_Combined_Definitions.pdf_tcm21-37252.pdf

Minnesota Statue Section 148.171
Chapter 148
Section 148.171 Definitions
"**Subd. 14. Practice of practical nursing**. The "practice of practical nursing" means the performance, with or without compensation of those services that incorporates caring for individual patients in all settings through nursing standards recognized by the board at the direction of a registered nurse, advanced practice registered nurse, or other licensed health care provider and includes, but is not limited to:

1) conducting a focused assessment of the health status of an individual patient through the collection and comparison of data to normal findings and the individual patient's current health status, and reporting changes and responses to interventions in an ongoing manner to a registered nurse or the appropriate licensed health care provider for delegated or assigned tasks or activities;

2) participating with other health care providers in the development and modification of a plan of care;

3) determining and implementing appropriate interventions within a nursing plan of care or when delegated or assigned by a registered nurse;

4) implementing interventions that are delegated, ordered, or prescribed by a licensed health care provider;

5) assigning nursing activities or tasks to other licensed practical nurses (LPNs);

6) assigning and monitoring nursing tasks or activities to unlicensed assistive personnel;

7) providing safe and effective nursing care delivery;

8) promoting a safe and therapeutic environment;

9) advocating for the best interests of individual patients;

10) assisting in the evaluation of responses to interventions;

11) collaborating and communicating with other health care providers;

12) providing health care information to individual patients;

13) providing input into the development of policies and procedures; and

14) accountability for the quality of care delivered, recognizing the limits of knowledge and experience; addressing situations beyond the nurse's competency; and performing to the level of education, knowledge, and skill ordinarily expected of an individual who has completed an approved practical nursing education program described in section 148.211, subdivision 1"(Minnesota Board of Nursing, 2013. P. 1–3)

Table 12.26   Mississippi

National Council of State Boards of Nursing (2017). Find your nurse practice act: Mississippi. Retrieved from https://www.ncsbn.org/npa.htm
Mississippi Board of Nursing (2010). Mississippi nursing practice law. Retrieved from http://www.msbn.ms.gov/Documents/NursingPracticeAct.pdf
Mississippi Nurse Practice Law
73-15-5 Definitions
"(5) The practice of nursing by a licensed practical nurse means the performance for compensation of services requiring basic knowledge of the biological, physical, behavioral, psychological and sociological sciences and of nursing procedures which do not require the substantial skill, judgment and knowledge required of a registered nurse. These services are performed under the direction of a registered nurse or a licensed physician or licensed dentist and utilize standardized procedures in the observation and care of the ill, injured and infirm; in the maintenance of health; in action to safeguard life and health; and in the administration of medications and treatments prescribed by any licensed physician or licensed dentist authorized by state law to prescribe. On a selected basis, and within safe limits, the role of the licensed practical nurse shall be expanded by the board under its rule-making authority to more complex procedures and settings commensurate with additional preparation and experience" (Mississippi Board of Nursing, 2010, p. 4)

Table 12.27   Missouri

National Council of State Boards of Nursing (2017). Find your nurse practice act: Missouri. Retrieved from https://www.ncsbn.org/npa.htm
Missouri Division of Professional Registration (2016). Missouri revised statutes. Chapter 335. Nurses. Retrieved from http://www.moga.mo.gov/mostatutes/ChaptersIndex/chaptIndex335.html
Missouri Practice Act and Regulations
Missouri State Board of Nursing
Chapter 335 Nurse Practice Act
335.016 Definitions
"(14) **'Practical nursing'**, the performance for compensation of selected acts for the promotion of health and in the care of persons who are ill, injured, or experiencing alterations in normal health processes. Such performance requires substantial specialized skill, judgment and knowledge. All such nursing care shall be given under the direction of a person licensed by a state regulatory board to prescribe medications and treatments or under the direction of a registered professional nurse. For the purposes of this chapter, the term **"direction"** shall mean guidance or supervision provided by a person licensed by a state regulatory board to prescribe medications and treatments or a registered professional nurse, including, but not limited to, oral, written, or otherwise communicated orders or directives for patient care. When practical nursing care is delivered pursuant to the direction of a person licensed by a state regulatory board to prescribe medications and treatments or under the direction of a registered professional nurse, such care may be delivered by a licensed practical nurse without direct physical oversight" (Missouri Division of Professional Registration, 2016, para. 14)

(continued)

Table 12.27 (continued)

335.017 Intravenous Fluids and Administration Requirements for Practical Nurses
"One of the selected acts which may be performed by persons licensed under the provisions of
this chapter as licensed practical nurses is the administration of intravenous fluid treatment. The
administration of intravenous fluid treatment may be performed only by licensed practical
nurses who have been instructed and trained in such procedures in a course of instruction
approved by the board. The board shall have the authority to adopt and revise rules and
regulations which limit and define the scope of intravenous fluid treatment which may be
performed by licensed practical nurses. Nothing herein shall be construed as prohibiting
administration of intravenous fluid treatment by registered professional nurses. The board shall
submit emergency rules to the secretary of state to implement the provisions of this section
within thirty days of December 15, 1983, and the board shall act promptly on applications of
organizations requesting approval of their course of instruction" (Missouri Division of
Professional Registration, 2016, para. 1)

335.099 "Licensed practical nurse, additional authorized acts. Any licensed practical nurse, as
defined in Section 335.016:
  (1) Who is an approved instructor for the level 1 medication aid program shall be qualified
      to teach the insulin administration course under Chapter 198
  (2) Shall be qualified to perform diabetic nail care and monthly on-site reviews of basic
      personal care recipients, as required by the Department of Social Services, of a resident
      of a residential care facility or assisted living facility, as defined in Chapter 198
  (3) Shall be qualified to perform dietary oversight, as required by the Department of Health
      and Senior Services, of a resident of a residential care facility or assisted living facility,
      as defined in Chapter 198" (Missouri Division of Professional Registration, 2016,
      para. 1)

Table 12.28 Montana

National Council of State Boards of Nursing (2017). Find your nurse practice act: Montana.
Retrieved from https://www.ncsbn.org/npa.htm

Montana Department of Labor and Industry (2015). Board of Nursing. Regulations. Title 37
Professions and Occupations. Chapter 8 Nursing. Retrieved from http://leg.mt.gov/bills/
mca_toc/37_8.htm

Title 37 Professions and Occupations
Chapter 8 Nursing
Part 1 General
Definitions
37-8-102. Definitions
  (8) (a) "Practice of practical nursing" means the performance of services requiring basic
      knowledge of the biological, physical, behavioral, psychological, and sociological sciences
      and of nursing procedures. The practice of practical nursing uses standardized procedures in
      the observation and care of the ill, injured, and infirm, in the maintenance of health, in
      action to safeguard life and health, and in the administration of medications and treatments
      prescribed by a physician, naturopathic physician, physician assistant, optometrist,
      advanced practice registered nurse, dentist, osteopath, or podiatrist authorized by state law
      to prescribe medications and treatments. These services are performed under the supervision
      of a registered nurse or a physician, naturopathic physician, physician assistant, optometrist,
      dentist, osteopath, or podiatrist authorized by state law to prescribe medications and
      treatments. (b) These services may include a charger nurse capacity in a long-term facility
      that provides skilled nursing care or intermediate nursing care as defined in 50-5-101, under
      general supervision of a RN
  (b) These services may include a charge nurse capacity in a long-term care facility that provides
      skilled nursing care or intermediate nursing care, as defined in 50-5-101, under the general
      supervision of a registered nurse" (Montana Department of Labor and Industry, 2015, para.
      8)

Table 12.29   Nebraska

National Council of State Boards of Nursing (2017). Find your nurse practice act: Nebraska. Retrieved from https://www.ncsbn.org/npa.htm

Nebraska Department of Health and Human Services (2012). Statutes relating to nurse practice act. Retrieved from http://dhhs.ne.gov/publichealth/Licensure/Documents/Nursing-NursePracticeAct.pdf

38-2209

"Licensed practitioner, defined. Licensed practitioner means a person lawfully authorized to prescribe medications or treatments" (Nebraska Department of Health and Human Services, 2012, p. 1)

38-2211

"Practice of nursing by a licensed practical nurse, defined:
  1) Practice of nursing by a licensed practical nurse means the assumption of responsibilities and accountability for nursing practice in accordance with knowledge and skills acquired through an approved program of practical nursing. A licensed practical nurse may function at the direction of a licensed practitioner or a registered nurse
  2) Such responsibilities and performances of acts must utilize procedures leading to predictable outcomes and must include, but not be limited to:
    a) Contributing to the assessment of the health status of individuals and groups
    b) Participating in the development and modification of a plan of care
    c) Implementing the appropriate aspects of the plan of care
    d) Maintaining safe and effective nursing care rendered directly or indirectly
    e) Participating in the evaluation of response to interventions
    f) Assigning and directing nursing interventions that may be performed by others and that do not conflict with the Nurse Practice Act" (Nebraska Department of Health and Human Services, 2012, p. 1)

Table 12.30   Nevada

National Council of State Boards of Nursing (2017). Find your nurse practice act: Nevada. Retrieved from https://www.ncsbn.org/npa.htm

Nevada State Board of Nursing (2017). Nurse practice act. Chapter 32 Nursing. Retrieved from https://www.leg.state.nv.us/NRS/NRS-632.html

NRS 632.017   Practice of Practical Nursing Defined

"Practice of practical nursing' means the performance of selected acts in the care of the ill, injured or infirm under the direction of a registered professional nurse, an advanced practice registered nurse, a licensed physician, a physician assistant licensed pursuant to chapter 630 or 633 of NRS, a licensed dentist or a licensed podiatric physician, not requiring the substantial specialized skill, judgment and knowledge required in professional nursing" (Nevada State Board of Nursing, 2017, para. 26)

Table 12.31 New Hampshire

National Council of State Boards of Nursing (2017). Find your nurse practice act: New Hampshire. Retrieved from https://www.ncsbn.org/npa.htm

New Hampshire Board of Nursing (2017). New Hampshire Statutes. Chapter 32-B: Nurse Practice Act. Retrieved from http://www.gencourt.state.nh.us/rsa/html/NHTOC/NHTOC-XXX-326-B.htm

Title 30 Occupations and Professions
Chapter 326B Nurse Practice Act
Section 326-B:13
326-B:13 Scope of Practice: Licensed Practical Nurse

I. "A LPN shall, with or without compensation or personal profit, practice under the supervision of an RN, APRN, licensed physician, or dentist. Such practice is guided by nursing standards established by the National Council of State Boards of Nursing and approved by the board and shall be limited to:

a) Collecting data and conducting focused nursing assessments of the health status of clients

b) Planning nursing care for clients with stable conditions

c) Participating in the development and modification of the comprehensive plan of care for all types of clients

d) Implementing appropriate aspects of the strategy of care within the LPN scope of practice

e) Participating in nursing care management through delegating, assigning, and directing nursing interventions that may be performed by others, including other LPNs that do not conflict with this chapter

f) Maintaining safe and effective nursing care rendered directly or indirectly

g) Promoting a safe and therapeutic environment

h) Participating in health teaching and counseling to promote, attain, and maintain the optimum health level of clients

i) Serving as an advocate for the client by communicating and collaborating with other health service personnel

j) Participating in the evaluation of client responses to interventions

k) Communicating and collaborating with other health-care professionals

l) Providing input into the development of policies and procedures

m) Other nursing services that require education and training prescribed by the board and in conformance with national nursing standards. Additional nursing services shall be commensurate with the LPN's experience, continuing education, and demonstrated LPN competencies

II. Each nurse is accountable to clients, the nursing profession, and the board for complying with the requirements of this chapter and the quality of nursing care rendered and for recognizing limits of knowledge and experience and planning for management of situations beyond the nurse's expertise

III. LPNs who have successfully completed the curriculum of a board-approved LPN intravenous therapy course may administer intravenous solutions under the direction of a physician or dentist or as delegated by an RN

IV. Any expansion of the scope of practice shall be adopted by the legislation in accordance with RSA 332-G:6" (New Hampshire Board of Nursing, 2017, Section 13)

Table 12.32   New Jersey

National Council of State Boards of Nursing (2017). Find your nurse practice act: New Jersey. Retrieved from https://www.ncsbn.org/npa.htm

New Jersey Division of Consumer Affairs (2017). New Jersey Board of Nursing. Statutes and Regulations

45:11-23 Definitions

"The practice of nursing as a licensed practical nurse is defined as performing tasks and responsibilities within the framework of casefinding; reinforcing the patient and family teaching program through health teaching, health counseling and provision of supportive and restorative care, under the direction of a registered nurse or licensed or otherwise legally authorized physician or dentist" (New Jersey Division of Consumer Affairs, 2017, p. 2)

Table 12.33   New Mexico

National Council of State Boards of Nursing (2017). Find your nurse practice act: New Mexico. Retrieved from https://www.ncsbn.org/npa.htm

New Mexico Board of Nursing (1978). New Mexico Nursing Practice Act, Chapter 61, Article 3. Retrieved from https://s3.amazonaws.com/realFile30f9bb9a-feed-462b-abce-56bd5dd949fa/7f352700-c71d-4d49-b4b3-53daf2a6b1d1?response-content-disposition=filename%3D%22NPA.pdf%22&response-content-type=application%2Fpdf&AWSAccessKeyId=AKIAIMZX6TNBAOLKC6MQ&Signature=S5zCQ60X9CIVbB3dbXdGhosQpmY%3D&Expires=1504255342

New Mexico Nurse Practice Act

Chapter 61, Article 3

61-3-3 Definitions

   I. "'Licensed practical nurse' means a nurse who practices licensed practical nursing and whose name and pertinent information are entered in the register of licensed practical nurses maintained by the board or a nurse who practices licensed practical nursing pursuant to a multistate licensure privilege as provided in the Nurse Licensure Compact

   II. 'Licensed practical nursing' means the practice of a directed scope of nursing requiring basic knowledge of the biological, physical, social, and behavioral sciences and nursing procedures, which practice is at the direction of a registered nurse, physician, or dentist licensed to practice in this state. This practice includes but is not limited to:

     1) Contributing to the assessment of the health status of individuals, families, and communities

     2) Participating in the development and modification of the plan of care

     3) Implementing appropriate aspects of the plan of care commensurate with education and verified competence

     4) Collaborating with other health-care professionals in the management of health care

     5) Participating in the evaluation of responses to interventions" (New Mexico Board of Nursing, 1978, p. 2)

Table 12.34 New York

National Council of State Boards of Nursing (2017). Find your nurse practice act: New York. Retrieved from https://www.ncsbn.org/npa.htm

NYSED.gov (2010). Education Law. Article 139, Nursing. Retrieved from http://www.op.nysed.gov/prof/nurse/article139.htm

Office of the Professions
Title 8 The Professions
Article 139 Nursing
§6901. Definitions

"The practice of nursing as a licensed practical nurse is defined as performing tasks and responsibilities within the framework of casefinding, health teaching, health counseling, and provision of supportive and restorative care under the direction of a registered professional nurse or licensed physician, dentist or other licensed health care provider legally authorized under this title and in accordance with the commissioner's regulations" (NYSED.gov, 2010, para. 6)

Table 12.35 North Carolina

National Council of State Boards of Nursing (2017). Find your nurse practice act: North Carolina. Retrieved from https://www.ncsbn.org/npa.htm

North Carolina Board of Nursing (2009). Nurse Practice Act. Retrieved from http://www.ncbon.com/myfiles/downloads/nursing-practice-act.pdf

North Carolina
Article 9a
Nursing Practice Act
90-171-20 Definitions

"(8) The 'practice of nursing by a licensed practical nurse' consists of the following seven components:

  a. Participating in the assessment of the patient's physical and mental health, including the patient's reaction to illnesses and treatment regimens.

  b. Recording and reporting the results of the nursing assessment.

  c. Participating in implementing the health care plan developed by the registered nurse and/or prescribed by any person authorized by State law to prescribe such a plan, by performing tasks assigned or delegated by and performed under the supervision or under orders or directions of a registered nurse, physician licensed to practice medicine, dentist, or other person authorized by State law to provide the supervision.

  d. Assigning or delegating nursing interventions to other qualified personnel under the supervision of the registered nurse.

  e. Participating in the teaching and counseling of patients as assigned by a registered nurse, physician, or other qualified professional licensed to practice in North Carolina.

  f. Reporting and recording the nursing care rendered and the patient's response to that care.

  g. Maintaining safe and effective nursing care, whether rendered directly or indirectly" (North Carolina Board of Nursing, 2009, p. 4)

Table 12.36 North Dakota

National Council of State Boards of Nursing (2017). Find your nurse practice act: North Dakota. Retrieved from https://www.ncsbn.org/npa.htm
North Dakota Board of Nursing (2017). Chapter 43-12.1 Nurse Practices Act. Retrieved from http://www.legis.nd.gov/cencode/t43c12-1.pdf#nameddest=43-12p1-02
North Dakota Century Code for Board of Nursing
Chapter 43-12.1 Nurse Practices Act
43-12.1-02 Definitions
"Licensed practical nurse" means an individual who holds a current license to practice in this state as a licensed practical nurse and who practices dependently under the supervision of a registered nurse, specialty practice registered nurse, advanced practice registered nurse, or licensed practitioner (North Dakota Board of Nursing, 2017, p. 1)
'Nurse' means an individual who is currently licensed as an advanced practice registered nurse, specialty practice registered nurse, registered nurse, or licensed practical nurse (North Dakota Board of Nursing, 2017, p. 1)
'Nursing' means the performance of acts utilizing specialized knowledge, skills, and abilities for people in a variety of settings. The term includes the following acts, which may not be deemed to include acts of medical diagnosis or treatment or the practice of medicine as defined in Chapter 43-17:
  a. The maintenance of health and prevention of illness
  b. Assessing and diagnosing human responses to actual or potential health problems
  c. Providing supportive and restorative care and nursing treatment, medication administration, health counseling and teaching, case finding, and referral of individuals who are ill, injured, or experiencing changes in the normal health processes
  d. Administration, teaching, supervision, delegation, and evaluation of health and nursing practices
  e. Collaboration with other health-care professionals in the implementation of the total health-care regimen and execution of the health-care regimen prescribed by a health-care practitioner licensed under the laws of this state" (North Dakota Board of Nursing, 2017, p. 1)

Table 12.37 Northern Mariana Islands

National Council of State Boards of Nursing (2017). Find your nurse practice act: North Mariana Islands. Retrieved from https://www.ncsbn.org/npa.htm
House of Representatives, Fourteenth Northern Marianas Commonwealth Legislature (2004). First Regular Session, An Act. Public Law No. 14-62. H.B. No. 14-7, SDI. Retrieved from http://www.cnmilaw.org/pdf/public_laws/14/pl14-62.pdf
Section 2304. Definitions and Scope
""Licensed practical/vocational nurse" means a person in the practice of nursing as a licensed practical/vocational nurse with a directed scope of nursing practice that shall include, but not limited to:
  1. Contributing to the health status of individuals and groups
  2. Participating in the development and modification of strategy of care
  3. Implementing the appropriate aspects of strategy of care as defined by the board
  4. Maintaining safe and effective nursing care rendered directly or indirectly
  5. Participating in the evaluation of responses to interventions
  6. Delegating nursing interventions to qualified others as provided in this chapter
The licensed practical/vocational nurse practices under the direction of the licensed registered nurse, licensed advanced practiced registered nurse, licensed physician, or licensed dentist in the performance of activities delegated by that health-care professional" (House of Representatives, Fourteenth Northern Marianas Commonwealth Legislature, 2004, p. 4–5)
"The 'Practice of Nursing' means assisting individuals or groups to maintain or attain optimal health, implementing a strategy of care to accomplish defined goals, and evaluating responses to care and treatment. This practice shall include, but not be limited to, initiating and maintaining comfort measures, promoting and supporting human functions and response, establishing an environment conducive to well-being, providing health counseling and teaching, and collaborating on certain aspects of the health regimen. This practice is based on understanding the human condition across the lifespan and the relationship of the individual within the environment" (House of Representatives, Fourteenth Northern Marianas Commonwealth Legislature, 2004, p. 5)

Table 12.38 Ohio

National Council of State Boards of Nursing (2017). Find your nurse practice act: Ohio. Retrieved from https://www.ncsbn.org/npa.htm

The Ohio Board of Nursing (2017). Chapter 4723.01 Nurses. Retrieved from http://codes.ohio. gov/orc/4723

4723.01 Nurse Definitions

(F) ""The practice of nursing as a licensed practical nurse" means providing to individuals and groups nursing care requiring the application of basic knowledge of the biological, physical, behavioral, social, and nursing sciences at the direction of a registered nurse or any of the following who is authorized to practice in this state: a physician, physician assistant, dentist, podiatrist, optometrist, or chiropractor. Such nursing care includes:

    1) Observation, patient teaching, and care in a diversity of health-care settings

    2) Contributions to the planning, implementation, and evaluation of nursing

    3) Administration of medications and treatments authorized by an individual who is authorized to practice in this state and is acting within the course of the individual's professional practice on the condition that the licensed practical nurse is authorized under section 4723.17 of the Revised Code to administer medications

    4) Administration to an adult of intravenous therapy authorized by an individual who is authorized to practice in this state and is acting within the course of the individual's professional practice, on the condition that the licensed practical nurse is authorized under section 4723.18 or 4723.181 of the Revised Code to perform intravenous therapy and performs intravenous therapy only in accordance with those sections

    5) Delegation of nursing tasks as directed by a registered nurse

    6) Teaching nursing tasks to licensed practical nurses and individuals to whom the licensed practical nurse is authorized to delegate nursing tasks as directed by a registered nurse" (The Ohio Board of Nursing, 2017, para. 1)

Chapter 4723-4 Standards of Practice Relative to Registered Nurse or Licensed Practical Nurse

4723-4-04 Standards Relating to Competent Practice as a Licensed Practical Nurse

    A. *"A licensed practical nurse shall function within the scope of practice of nursing for a licensed practical nurse as set forth in division (F) of Section 4723.01 of the Revised Code and the rules of the board*

    B. *A licensed practical nurse shall maintain current knowledge of the duties, responsibilities, and accountabilities for safe nursing practice*

    C. *A licensed practical nurse shall demonstrate competence and accountability in all areas of practice in which the nurse is engaged which includes, but is not limited to, the following*:

1. Consistent performance of all aspects of nursing care

2. Recognition, referral or consultation, and intervention, when a complication arises

    D. A licensed practical nurse may provide nursing care in accordance with division (F) of Section 4723.01 of the Revised Code that is beyond basic preparation for a licensed practical nurse provided:

1. The nurse obtains education that emanates from a recognized body of knowledge relative to the nursing care to be provided

2. The nurse demonstrates knowledge, skills, and abilities necessary to perform the nursing care

3. The nurse maintains documentation satisfactory to the board of meeting the requirements set forth in paragraphs (D)(1) and (D)(2) of this rule

4. When the nursing care to be provided according to division (F)(3) of Section 4723.01 of the Revised Code, the nurse has a specific current valid order or direction from an individual who is authorized to practice in this state and is acting within the course of the individual's professional practice

5. The nursing care does not involve a function or procedure that is prohibited by any other law or rule

Table 12.38   (continued)

E. A licensed practical nurse shall, in a timely manner:

1. Implement any order or direction for a patient unless the licensed practical nurse believes or should have the reason to believe that the order or direction is:
a) Inaccurate
b) Not properly authorized
c) Not current or valid
d) Harmful or potentially harmful to a patient
e) Contraindicated by other documented information

2. Clarify any order or direction for a patient when the licensed practical nurse believes or should have the reason to believe that the order or direction is:
a) Inaccurate
b) Not properly authorized
c) Not current or valid
d) Harmful or potentially harmful to a patient
e) Contraindicated by other documented information

F. When clarifying an order or direction, the licensed practical nurse shall, in a timely manner:

1. Consult with an appropriate licensed practitioner or directing registered nurse
2. Notify the ordering practitioner or directing registered nurse when the licensed practical nurse makes the decision not to follow the order or direction or administer the medication or treatment as prescribed
3. Document that the practitioner or directing registered nurse was notified of the decision not to follow the direction or order or administer the medication or treatment, including the reason for not doing so
4. Take any other action needed to assure the safety of the patient

G. A licensed practical nurse shall, in a timely manner, report to and consult as necessary with other nurses or other members of the health-care team and make referrals as necessary

H. A licensed practical nurse shall maintain the confidentiality of patient information obtained in the course of nursing practice. The licensed practical nurse shall communicate patient information with other members of the health-care team for health-care purposes only, shall access patient information only for purposes of patient care or for otherwise fulfilling the nurse's assigned job responsibilities, and shall not disseminate patient information for purposes other than patient care or for otherwise fulfilling the nurse's assigned job responsibilities, through social media, texting, emailing, or any other form of communication

I. To the maximum extent feasible, identifiable patient health-care information shall not be disclosed by a licensed practical nurse unless the patient has consented to the disclosure of identifiable patient health-care information. A licensed practical nurse shall report individually identifiable patient information without written consent in limited circumstances only and in accordance with an authorized law, rule, or other recognized legal authority

J. When a licensed practical nurse is directed to observe, advise, instruct, or evaluate the performance of a nursing task, the licensed practical nurse shall use acceptable standards of safe nursing care as a basis for that observation, advice, instruction, teaching, or evaluation and shall communicate information that is consistent with acceptable standards of safe nursing care" (The Ohio Board of Nursing, 2017, para. 3)

(continued)

Table 12.38   (continued)

4723-4-08 Standards for Applying the Nursing Process as a Licensed Practical Nurse
  A. "The licensed practical nurse shall contribute to the nursing process in the practice of
     nursing as set forth in division (F) of Section 4723.01 of the Revised Code and in the rules
     of the board. The nursing process is cyclical in nature so that the nurse's actions respond
     to the patient's changing status throughout the process. The licensed practical nurse is
     directed in providing nursing care by the established nursing plan. The following
     standards shall be used by a licensed practical nurse in utilization of the nursing process:
  1. Contribution to assessment of patient health status:The licensed practical nurse shall
     contribute to the nursing assessment of the patient. The licensed practical nurse shall, in an
     accurate and timely manner:
  a. Collect and document objective and subjective data related to the patient's health status
  b. Report objective and subjective data to the directing registered nurse or health-care provider
     and other members of the health-care team
  2. Planning:The licensed practical nurse shall, in an accurate and timely manner:
  a. Contribute to the development, maintenance, or modification of the nursing component of the
     care plan
  b. Communicate the nursing plan of care and all authorized modifications of the plan to
     members of the health-care team
  3. ImplementationThe licensed practical nurse shall, in an accurate and timely manner,
     implement the nursing plan of care, which may include:
  a. Providing nursing interventions
  b. Collecting and reporting patient data as directed
  c. Administering medications and treatments prescribed by an individual who is authorized to
     practice in this state and is acting within the course of the individual's professional practice
  d. Providing basic nursing care as directed by a registered nurse, advanced practice registered
     nurse, or licensed physician, dentist, optometrist, chiropractor, or podiatrist
  e. Collaborating with other nurses and other members of the health-care team
  f. Delegating nursing tasks as directed, including medication administration, only in accordance
     with Chapters 4723-13, 4723-23, 4723-26, or 4723-27 of the Administrative Code
  4. Contributing to evaluation:The licensed practical nurse shall, in an accurate and timely
     manner:
  a. Contribute to the evaluation of the patient's response to nursing interventions
  b. Document the patient's responses to nursing interventions
  c. Communicate the patient's responses to nursing interventions to the directing registered
     nurse or health-care provider and members of the health-care team
  d. Contribute to the reassessment of the patient's health status and to the modifications of any
     aspect of the nursing plan of care as set forth in this rule" (The Ohio Board of Nursing, 2017,
     para. 7)

Table 12.39 Oklahoma

National Council of State Boards of Nursing (2017). Find your nurse practice act: Oklahoma. Retrieved from https://www.ncsbn.org/npa.htm

Oklahoma Board of Nursing (2016). Oklahoma Nursing Practice Act. Retrieved from http://nursing.ok.gov/actwp16.pdf

Oklahoma Nursing Practice Act

§ 567.3a. Definitions

"'Licensed practical nursing' means the practice of nursing under the supervision or direction of a registered nurse, licensed physician, or dentist. This directed scope of nursing practice includes but is not limited to:

    a. Contributing to the assessment of the health status of individuals and groups

    b. Participating in the development and modification of the plan of care

    c. Implementing the appropriate aspects of the plan of care

    d. Delegating such tasks as may safely be performed by others, consistent with educational preparation and that do not conflict with the Oklahoma Nursing Practice Act

    e. Providing safe and effective nursing care rendered directly or indirectly

    f. Participating in the evaluation of responses to interventions

    g. Teaching basic nursing skills and related principles

    h. Performing additional nursing procedures in accordance with knowledge and skills acquired through education beyond nursing preparation

    i. Delegating those nursing tasks as defined in the rules of the board that may be performed by an advanced unlicensed assistive person" (Oklahoma Board of Nursing, 2016, p. 4)

Table 12.40 Oregon

National Council of State Boards of Nursing (2017). Find your nurse practice act: Oregon. Retrieved from https://www.ncsbn.org/npa.htm

Oregon State Board of Nursing (2017). Standards and scope of practice for the Licensed Practical Nurse and Registered Nurse. Retrieved from http://arcweb.sos.state.or.us/pages/rules/oars_800/oar_851/851_045.html

851-045-0050

Scope of Practice Standards for Licensed Practical Nurses

1. "The board recognizes that the LPN has a supervised practice that occurs at the clinical direction and under the clinical supervision of the RN or LIP who have authority to make changes in the plan of care and encompasses a variety of roles, including, but not limited to:

    a. Provision of client care

    b. Supervision of others in the provision of care

    c. Participation in the development and implementation of health-care policy

    d. Participation in nursing research

    e. Teaching health-care providers and prospective health-care providers

2. Standards related to the LPN's responsibility for ethical practice, accountability for services provided, and competency. The LPN shall:

    a. Base LPN practice on current nursing science, other sciences, and the humanities

    b. Be knowledgeable of the statutes and regulations governing LPN practice and practice within those legal boundaries

    c. Be knowledgeable of the professional nursing practice standards applicable to LPN practice and adhere to those standards

    d. Demonstrate honesty, integrity, and professionalism in the practice of licensed practical nursing

    e. Be accountable for individual LPN actions

    f. Maintain competency in one's LPN practice role

    g. Maintain documentation of the method that competency was acquired and maintained

    h. Accept only LPN assignments that are within one's individual scope of practice

(continued)

Table 12.40 (continued)

i. Recognize and respect a client's autonomy, dignity, and choice

j. Accept responsibility for notifying employer of an ethical objection to the provision of a specific nursing intervention

k. Ensure unsafe nursing practice is addressed immediately

l. Ensure unsafe practice and unsafe practice conditions are reported to the appropriate regulatory agency

m. Protect confidential client information and only share information in a manner that is consistent with current law

3. Standards related to the LPN's responsibility for nursing practice. Applying practical nursing knowledge, at the clinical direction and under the clinical supervision of the RN or LIP, the LPN shall:

a. Conduct focused assessments by:

A. Collecting data through observations, examinations, interviews, and records in an accurate and timely manner as appropriate to the client's health-care needs and context of care

B. Validating data by utilizing available resources, including interactions with the client and health-care team members

C. Distinguishing abnormal from normal data, sorting, selecting, recording, and reporting the data discrepancies to the supervising RN or supervising LIP

D. Identifying potentially inaccurate, incomplete, or missing data and reporting as needed

E. Recognizing signs and symptoms of deviation from current health status

F. Evaluating data to identify problems or risks presented by the client

b. Select reasoned conclusions that communicate client problems or risks

c. Contribute to the development of a comprehensive plan of care or develop a focused plan of care. This includes:

A. Identifying priorities in the plan of care

B. Setting measurable outcomes in collaboration with the client

C. Selecting appropriate nursing interventions as established by the RN or consistent with the LIP's plan of care

d. Implement the plan of care

e. Evaluate client responses to nursing interventions, progress toward measurable outcomes, and communicate such to appropriate members of the health-care team

4. Standards related to the LPN's responsibility to assign and supervise care. At the clinical direction and under the clinical supervision of the RN or LIP, the LPN:

a. May assign to a LPN, nursing interventions that fall within LPN scope of practice and that the licensee receiving the assignment possesses the competency to perform safely

b. May assign to the CNA and CMA the duties identified within Chapter 851 Division 63 that the certificate holder possesses the competency to perform safely

c. May assign to the UAP work the UAP is authorized to perform within the practice setting and that the UAP possesses the competency to perform safely

d. Shall ensure the assignment matches client service need

e. Shall provide clinical supervision of the LPN, CNA, CMA, and UAP to whom an assignment possesses been made:

A. Provides supervision per the context of care

B. Ensures documentation of supervision activities occurs per the context of the assignment

C. Evaluates the effectiveness of the assignment

D. Reports effectiveness of assignment to the supervising RN or supervising LIP

f. Shall revise the assignment as directed by the supervising RN or supervising LIP

g. Prior to making an assignment, the LPN is responsible to know the duties, activities, or procedures the recipient of the assignment is authorized to perform within the setting

5. Standards related to the LPN's responsibility for client advocacy. The LPN shall:

a. Advocate for the client's right to receive appropriate care, including client-centered care and end-of-life care, that is respectful of the client's needs, choices, and dignity

Table 12.40 (continued)

b. Intervene on behalf of the client to identify changes in health status; to protect, promote, and optimize health; and to alleviate suffering

c. Advocate for the client's right to receive appropriate and accurate information

d. Communicate client's choices, concerns, and special needs to the supervising RN or supervising LIP and to other members of the health-care team

e. Protect the client's right to participate or decline to participate in research

6. Standards related to the LPN's responsibility for collaboration with the health-care team. The LPN shall:

a. Function as a member of the health-care team

b. Collaborate in the development, implementation, and evaluation of an integrated plan of care appropriate to the context of care

c. Demonstrate a knowledge of health-care team members' roles

d. Communicate with the supervising RN or supervising LIP and other relevant health-care team members regarding the plan of care

e. Make referrals as directed in a timely manner and follow up on referrals made

7. Standards related to the LPN's responsibility for the environment of care. The LPN shall:

a. Promote and advocate for an environment conducive to safety

b. Identify safety and environmental concerns, take action to address those concerns, and report to the supervising RN or supervising LIP

8. Standards related to the LPN's responsibility for leadership and quality of care. The LPN shall:

a. Identify factors that affect the quality of nursing service delivery and report to the supervising RN or LIP

b. Implement policies, protocols, and guidelines that are pertinent to nursing service delivery

c. Contribute to the development and implementation of policies, protocols, and guidelines that are pertinent to the practice of nursing and to health services delivery

d. Participate in quality improvement initiatives and activities within the practice setting

e. Participate in the development and mentoring of new licensees, nursing colleagues, students, and members of the health-care team

9. Standards related to the LPN's responsibility for health promotion and teaching. At the clinical direction and under the clinical supervision of the RN or LIP, the LPN may participate in the development, implementation, and evaluation of teaching plans appropriate to the context of care that address the learner's learning needs, readiness to learn, and ability to learn

10. Standards related to the LPN's responsibility for cultural responsiveness. The LPN shall:

a. Apply a basic knowledge of cultural diversity

b. Recognize and respect the cultural values, beliefs, and customs of the client" (Oregon State Board of Nursing, 2017, para. 4)

Table 12.41 Pennsylvania

National Council of State Boards of Nursing (2017). Find your nurse practice act: Pennsylvania. Retrieved from https://www.ncsbn.org/npa.htm

Pennsylvania Department of State (2012). Board Laws and Regulations. Chapter 21. State Board of Nursing. Subchapter B. Practical Nursing. Retrieved from http://www.pacode.com/secure/data/049/chapter21/subchapBtoc.html

Pennsylvania

Chapter B Practical Nurses

21-145 Functions of the LPN

"The LPN is prepared to function as a member of the health-care team by exercising sound nursing judgment based on preparation, knowledge, experience in nursing, and competency. The LPN participates in the planning, implementation, and evaluation of nursing care using focused assessment in settings where nursing takes place

a. A LPN shall communicate with a licensed professional nurse and the patient's health-care team members to seek guidance when:i. The patient care needs exceed the LPN scope of practiceii. The patient care needs surpass LPN knowledge, skills, or abilityiii. The patient condition deteriorates, there is a significant change in condition, the patient is not responding to therapy, the patient becomes unstable, or the patient needs immediate assistance

   1. A LPN shall obtain instruction and supervision if implementing new or unfamiliar nursing practices or procedures

   2. A LPN shall follow the written, established policies and procedures of the facility that are consistent with the act

b. The LPN administers medication and carries out therapeutic treatment ordered for the patient in accordance with the following:

   1. The LPN may accept a written order for medication and therapeutic treatment from a practitioner authorized by law and by facility policy to issue orders for medical and therapeutic measures

   2. The LPN may accept oral order if the following conditions are met:

      i. The practitioner issuing the oral order is authorized by law and by facility policy to issue oral orders for medical and therapeutic measures

      ii. The LPN has received instruction and training in accepting an oral order in an approved nursing education program or has received instruction and training in accepting an oral order in accordance with established policies and protocols of facility

      iii. The policy of the facility permits LPN to accept an oral order

      iv. The regulations governing the facility permit a LPN to accept an oral order

   3. The LPN shall question any order which is perceived as unsafe or contraindicated for the patient of which is not clear and shall raise the issue with the ordering practitioner. If the ordering practitioner is not available, the LPN shall raise issue with a RN or other responsible person in a manner consistent with protocol or policies of facility

   4. The LPN may not accept an oral order which is not within scope of functions permitted by this section or which LPN does not understand

   5. An oral order accepted by LPN shall be immediately transcribed by LPN in the proper place on the medical record of patient. The transcription shall include the prescriber's name, the date, the time of acceptance of the oral order, and full signature of LPN accepting oral order. The countersignature of ordering practitioner shall be obtained in accordance with applicable regulations of the Department of Health governing the licensed facility

c. The LPN participates in the development, revision, and implementation of policies and procedures designed to insure comfort and safety of patients in collaboration with other health-care personnel

Table 12.41 (continued)

d. The board recognizes codes of behavior as developed by appropriate practical nursing associations as criteria for assuring safe and effective practice

e. The LPN may administer immunizing agents and do skin testing only if the following conditions are met:

1. The LPN has received and satisfactorily completed board-approved educational program which requires study and supervised clinical practice intended to provide training necessary for administering immunizing agents and for performing skin testing

2. A written order has been issued by a licensed physician pertaining to individual patient or group of patients

3. Written policies and procedures under which LPN may administer immunizing agents and do skin testing have been established by the committee representing nurses, physicians, and the administration of the agency or institution employing or having jurisdiction over the LPN. A current copy of policies and procedures shall be provided to LPN at least once every 12 months. The policies and procedures shall provide for:

   i. Identification of immunizing and skin testing agents which LPN may administer
   ii. Determination of contraindications for administration of specific immunizing and skin testing agents
   iii. The listing, identification, description, and explanation of principles, including technical and clinical indications, necessary for the identification and treatment of possible adverse reactions
   iv. Instruction and supervised practice required to insure competency in administering immunizing and skin testing agents

f. A LPN may perform only the IV therapy functions for which the LPN possesses the knowledge, skill, and ability to perform in a safe manner, except as limited under 21.145a (relating to prohibited acts), and only under supervision as required under paragraph (1):

1. A LPN may initiate and maintain IV therapy only under the direction and supervision of licensed professional nurse or health-care provider authorized to issue orders for medical therapeutic or corrective measures (such as CRNP, physician, PA, podiatrist, or dentist)

2. Prior to initiation of IV therapy, LPN shall:
   i. Verify order and identification of patient
   ii. Identify allergies, fluid, and medication compatibilities
   iii. Monitor patient's circulatory system and infusion site
   iv. Inspect all equipment
   v. Instruction patient regarding risk and complication of therapy

3. Maintenance of IV therapy by LPN shall include ongoing observation and focused assessment of patient, monitoring the IV site, and maintaining equipment

4. For patient whose condition is determined by LPN supervisor to be stable and predictable and rapid change is not anticipated, the supervisor may supervise the LPN provision of IV therapy by physical presence or electronic communication. If supervision is provided by electronic communication, the LPN shall have access to assistance readily available.

5. In the following cases, a LPN may provide IV therapy only when LPN supervisor is physically present in immediate vicinity of LPN and immediately available to intervene in care of patient:
   i. When a patient's condition is critical, fluctuating, unstable, or unpredictable
   ii. When patient has developed signs and symptoms of IV catheter-related infection, venous thrombosis, or central line catheter occlusion
   iii. When a patient is receiving hemodialysis

g. A LPN who has met the education and training requirements of 21.145b (relating to IV therapy curriculum requirements) may perform the following IV therapy functions, except as limited under 21.145a and only under supervision as required under subsection (f):

(continued)

Table 12.41 (continued)

1. Adjustment of flow rate on IV infusions
2. Observation and reporting of subjective and objective signs of adverse reactions to any IV administration and initiation of appropriate interventions
3. Administration of IV fluids and medications
4. Observation of IV insertion site and performance of insertion site care
5. Performance of maintenance. Maintenance includes dressing changes, IV tubing changes, and saline or heparin flushes
6. Discontinuance of a medication or fluid infusion, including infusion devices
7. Conversion of continuous infusion to an intermittent infusion
8. Insertion or removal of peripheral short catheter
9. Maintenance, monitoring, and discontinuance of blood, blood components, and plasma volume expanders
10. Administration of solutions to maintain patency of IV access device via direct push or bolus route
11. Maintenance and discontinuance of IV medications and fluids given via a patient-controlled administration system
12. Administration and maintenance of discontinuation of parental nutrition and fat emulsion solutions
13. Collection of blood specimens from IV access device" (Pennsylvania Department of State, 2012, para. 15)

Table 12.42 Rhode Island

National Council of State Boards of Nursing (2017). Find your nurse practice act: Rhode Island. Retrieved from https://www.ncsbn.org/npa.htm

State of Rhode Island Department of Health (2017). Title 5. Businesses and Professions. Chapter 5-34. Nurses. Section 5-34-3. Retrieved from http://webserver.rilin.state.ri.us/Statutes/TITLE5/5-34/5-34-3.HTM

Rhode Island
Title 5 Businesses and Professions
Chapter 5-34 Nurses
5-34-1.1 Title of Act
This act shall be known and may be cited as "the Rhode Island Nurse Practice Act"
5-34-3 Definitions
"As used in this chapter:

(12) "Practical nursing" is practiced by LPNs. It is an integral part of nursing based on a knowledge and skill level commensurate with education. It includes promotion, maintenance, and restoration of health and utilizes standardized procedures leading to predictable outcomes that are in accord with professional nurse regimen under the direction of RN. In situations where RNs are not employed, the LPN functions under the direction of a licensed physician, dentist, podiatrist, or other licensed health-care providers authorized by law to prescribe. Each LPN is responsible for nursing care rendered" (State of Rhode Island Department of Health, 2017, para. 12)

Table 12.43 South Carolina

National Council of State Boards of Nursing (2017). Find your nurse practice act: South Carolina. Retrieved from https://www.ncsbn.org/npa.htm

South Carolina Legislature (2005). South Carolina Code of Laws, Unannotated. Chapter 33, Nurses, Article 1, Nurse Practice Act. Retrieved from http://www.scstatehouse.gov/code/t40c033.php

South Carolina Code of Laws Unannotated

Title 40 - Professions and Occupations

Chapter 33 Nurses

Article 1 Nurse Practice Act

Section 40-33-20 Definitions

"(47) Practice of Practical nursing means the performance of health care acts that require knowledge, judgment and skill and must be performed under supervision of an advanced practice RN, RN, licensed physician, licensed dentist, or other practitioner authorized by law to supervise LPN practice. The practice of Practical nursing includes, but is not limited to:

a) Collecting health care data to assist in planning care of persons;

b) Administering and delivering medications and treatments as prescribed by an authorized licensed provider;

c) Implementing nursing interventions and tasks;

d) Providing basic teaching for health promotion and maintenance;

e) Assisting in evaluation of responses to interventions;

f) Providing for maintenance of safe and effective nursing care rendered directly or indirectly;

g) Participating with other health care providers in planning and delivering of health care;

h) Delegating nursing tasks to qualified others;

i) Performing additional acts that require special education and training and that are approved by board including, but not limited to, IV therapy and other specific nursing acts and functioning as a charge nurse" (South Carolina Legislature, 2005, Section 40-33-20, para. 48)

Table 12.44 South Dakota

National Council of State Boards of Nursing (2017). Find your nurse practice act: South Dakota. Retrieved from https://www.ncsbn.org/npa.htm

South Dakota Department of Health (2012). South Dakota Board of Nursing. Nurses Practice Act. Chapter 36-9. Retrieved from http://www.sdlegislature.gov/Statutes/Codified_Laws/DisplayStatute.aspx?Type=Statute&Statute=36-9-4

South Dakota

Chapter 36-9 Registered and Practical Nurses

36-9-4

"Practice of licensed practical nurse. A licensed practical nurse practices under the supervision of a registered nurse, advanced practice registered nurse, licensed physician, or other health care provider authorized by the state. A licensed practical nurse is guided by nursing standards established or recognized by the board and includes:

1) Collecting data and conducting a focused nursing assessment of the health status of a patient;

2) Participating with other health care providers in the development and modification of the patient-centered health care plan;

3) Implementing nursing interventions within a patient-centered health care plan;

4) Assisting in the evaluation of responses to interventions;

5) Providing for the maintenance of safe and effective nursing care rendered directly or indirectly;

6) Advocating for the best interest of the patient;

7) Communicating and collaborating with patients and members of the health care team;

8) Assisting with health counseling and teaching;

9) Delegating and assigning nursing interventions to implement the plan of care; and

10) Other acts that require education and training consistent with professional standards as prescribed by the board, by rules promulgated pursuant to chapter 1-26, and commensurate with the licensed practical nurse's education, demonstrated competence, and experience" (South Dakota Department of Health, 2012, para. 1)

Table 12.45 Tennessee

National Council of State Boards of Nursing (2017). Find your nurse practice act: Tennessee. Retrieved from https://www.ncsbn.org/npa.htm

Tennessee Department of Health (2015). Rules of the Tennessee Board of Nursing. Chapter 1000-02, Rules and Regulations of Licensed Practical Nurses. Retrieved from http://share. tn.gov/sos/rules/1000/1000-02.20150622.pdf

Chapter 1000-02

Rules and Regulations of Licensed Practical Nurses

1000-02-.14 Standards of Nursing Competence

"The Board requires all nurses to document evidence of competence in their current practice role. The Board believes that the individual nurse is responsible for maintaining and demonstrating competence in the practice role whether the recipient of the nursing intervention is the individual, family, community, nursing staff, nursing student body, or other.

1) Standards of Nursing Practice for the Licensed Practical Nurse.

   a) Standards Related to the Licensed Practical Nurse's Contribution to and Responsibility for the Nursing Process - The Licensed Practical Nurse shall:

      1. Contribute to the nursing assessment by collecting, reporting and recording objective and subjective data in an accurate and timely manner.

      2. Participate in the development of the plan of care/action in consultation with a Registered Nurse.

      3. Participate in the assisting and giving of safe direct care.

      4. Participate in establishing and maintaining a therapeutic nurse/client relationship.

      5. Seek resources for patients/clients with cultural, physical or language barriers.

      6. Contribute to the evaluation of the responses of individuals or groups to nursing interventions and participate in revising the plan of care where appropriate.

      7. Communicate accurately in writing and orally with recipients of nursing care and other professionals.

   b) Standards Relating to the Licensed Practical Nurse's Responsibilities as a Member of the Health Team - The Licensed Practical Nurse shall:

      1. Integrate knowledge of the statutes and regulations governing nursing and function within the legal and ethical boundaries of practical nursing practice.

      2. Demonstrate personal responsibility for individual nursing actions and currency of competence.

      3. Consult with Registered Nurses and/or other health team members and seek guidance as necessary.

      4. Identify practice abilities and limitations and obtain instruction and supervision as necessary when implementing essential functions of the practice role.

      5. Report unsafe practice and unsafe practice conditions to recognized legal authorities and to the Board where appropriate.

      6. Conduct practice without discrimination on the basis of age, race, religion, sex, sexual preference, national origin, language, handicap, or disease.

      7. Demonstrate respect for the dignity and rights of clients regardless of social or economic status, personal attributes or nature of health problems.

      8. Protect confidential information, unless obligated by law to disclose such information.

      9. Demonstrate respect for the property of clients, family, significant others, and the employer.

      10. Participate in activities designed to improve health care delivery in any setting.

      11. Exhibit ethical behavior" (Tennessee Department of Health, 2015, p. 28–29)

Table 12.46 Texas

National Council of State Boards of Nursing (2017). Find your nurse practice act: Texas. Retrieved from https://www.ncsbn.org/npa.htm

Texas Board of Nursing (2013). Nursing Practice Act, Nursing peer review, and nurse licensure compact. Texas occupations code and statutes regulating the practice of nursing. Retrieved from http://www.bon.state.tx.us/pdfs/law_rules_pdfs/nursing_practice_act_pdfs/npa2013.pdf

Texas Nursing Practice Act,
Nursing Peer Review Act, and Nurse Licensure Compact
Sec. 301.002. Definitions

(4) "'Nursing' means professional or vocational nursing

(5) 'Vocational nursing' means a directed scope of nursing practice, including the performance of an act that requires specialized judgment and skill, the proper performance of which is based on knowledge and application of the principles of biological, physical, and social science as acquired by a completed course in an approved school of vocational nursing. The term does not include acts of medical diagnosis or the prescription of therapeutic or corrective measures. Vocational nursing involves:

(A) Collecting data and performing focused nursing assessments of the health status of an individual

(B) Participating in the planning of the nursing care needs of an individual

(C) Participating in the development and modification of the nursing care plan

(D) Participating in health teaching and counseling to promote, attain, and maintain the optimum health level of an individual

(E) Assisting in the evaluation of an individual's response to a nursing intervention and the identification of an individual's needs

(F) Engaging in other acts that require education and training, as prescribed by board rules and policies, commensurate with the nurse's experience, continuing education, and demonstrated competency" (Texas Board of Nursing, 2013, p. 1)

Table 12.47 Utah

National Council of State Boards of Nursing (2017). Find your nurse practice act: Utah. Retrieved from https://www.ncsbn.org/npa.htm

Utah Division of Occupational and Professional Licensing (2016). Chapter 31b, Nurse Practice Act. Retrieved from https://le.utah.gov/xcode/Title58/Chapter31b/58-31b.html

Index Utah Code
Title 58 Occupations and Professions
Chapter 31b Nurse Practice Act
Part 1 General Provisions
Section 102 Definitions

(16) "'Practice of practical nursing' means the performance of nursing acts in the generally recognized scope of practice of LPN as defined by rule and as provided in this subsection (16) by a person licensed under this chapter as a LPN and under the direction of a RN, licensed physician, or other specified health-care professional as defined by rule. Practical nursing acts include:

a) Contributing to assessment of health status of individuals and groups

b) Participating in the development and modification of the strategy of care

c) Implementing appropriate aspects of the strategy of care

d) Maintaining safe and effective nursing care rendered to a patient directly or indirectly

e) Participating in the evaluation of responses to interventions" (Utah Division of Occupational and Professional Licensing, 2016, p. 3)

Table 12.48 Vermont

National Council of State Boards of Nursing (2017). Find your nurse practice act: Vermont. Retrieved from https://www.ncsbn.org/npa.htm

Vermont Secretary of State (2017). Statutes and Rules. Title 26: Professions and Occupations. Chapter 28: Nursing. Subchapter 1: General Provisions. Retrieved from http://legislature. vermont.gov/statutes/section/26/028/01572

Title 26: Professions and Occupations
Chapter 28: Nursing
Subchapter 1: General Provisions
1572 Definitions
(3) "'Licensed practical nursing' means a directed scope of nursing practice that includes:
   A. Contributing to the assessment of the health status of individuals and groups
   B. Participating in the development and modification of the strategy of care
   C. Implementing the appropriate aspects of the strategy of care as defined by the board
   D. Maintaining safe and effective nursing care rendered directly or indirectly
   E. Participating in the evaluation of responses to interventions
   F. Delegating nursing interventions that may be performed by others and that do not conflict with this chapter
   G. Functioning at the direction of a RN, advanced practice RN, licensed physician, or licensed dentist in performance of activities delegated by that health-care professional" (Vermont Secretary of State, 2017, para. 3)

Table 12.49 Virginia

National Council of State Boards of Nursing (2017). Find your nurse practice act: Virginia. Retrieved from https://www.ncsbn.org/npa.htm

Virginia Board of Nursing (2017). Chapter 30 of Title 54.1 of the Code of Virginia Nursing. Retrieved from http://www.dhp.virginia.gov/nursing/nursing_laws_regs.htm

Chapter 30 of Title 54.1 of the Code of Virginia Nursing
54.1-3000 Definitions
"'Practical nursing' or 'licensed practical nursing' means the performance for compensation of selected nursing acts in the care of individuals or groups who are ill, injured, or experiencing changes in normal health processes; in the maintenance of health; in the prevention of illness or disease; or, subject to such regulations as the board may promulgate, in the teaching of those who are or will be nurse aides. Practical nursing or licensed practical nursing requires knowledge, judgment, and skill in nursing procedures gained through prescribed education. Practical nursing or licensed practical nursing is performed under the direction or supervision of a licensed medical practitioner, a professional nurse, registered nurse or registered professional nurse, or other licensed health professional authorized by regulations of the board" (Virginia Board of Nursing, 2017, p. 4–5)

Table 12.50 Washington

National Council of State Boards of Nursing (2017). Find your nurse practice act: Washington. Retrieved from https://www.ncsbn.org/npa.htm

Washington State Department of Health (2012). Chapter 18.79 RCW, Nursing Care. Retrieved from http://app.leg.wa.gov/RCW/default.aspx?cite=18.79.060

Chapter 18.79 RCW

Nursing Care

RCW 18.79.060

"LPN Practice" Defined: Exceptions

"'Licensed practical nursing practice' means the performance of services requiring the knowledge, skill, and judgment necessary for carrying out selected aspects of the designated nursing regimen under the direction and supervision of a licensed physician and surgeon, dentist, osteopathic physician and surgeon, physician assistant, osteopathic physician assistant, podiatric physician and surgeon, advanced registered nurse practitioner, registered nurse, or midwife. Nothing in this section prohibits a person from practicing a profession for which a license has been issued under the laws of this state or specifically authorized by any other law of the state of Washington. This section does not prohibit the nursing care of the sick, without compensation, by an unlicensed person who does not hold himself or herself out to be a licensed practical nurse" (Washington State Department of Health, 2012, para. 1)

RCW 18.79.270

Licensed Practical Nurse: Activities Allowed

"A licensed practical nurse under his or her license may perform nursing care, as that term is usually understood, of the ill, injured, or infirm, and in the course thereof may, under the direction of a licensed physician and surgeon, osteopathic physician and surgeon, dentist, naturopathic physician, podiatric physician and surgeon, physician assistant, osteopathic physician assistant, advanced registered nurse practitioner, or midwife acting under the scope of his or her license, or at the direction and under the supervision of a registered nurse, administer drugs, medications, treatments, tests, injections, and inoculations, whether or not the piercing of tissues is involved and whether or not a degree of independent judgment and skill is required, when selected to do so by one of the licensed practitioners designated in this section, or by a registered nurse who need not be physically present; if the order given is reduced to writing within a reasonable time and made a part of the patient's record. Such direction must be for acts within the scope of licensed practical nurse practice" (Washington State Department of Health, 2012, para. 1)

Table 12.51 West Virginia

National Council of State Boards of Nursing (2017). Find your nurse practice act: West Virginia. Retrieved from https://www.ncsbn.org/npa.htm

West Virginia Legislature (2016). Chapter 30 Professions and Occupations, Article 7A Practical Nurses. Retrieved from http://www.legis.state.wv.us/WVCODE/Code. cfm?chap=30&art=7A#07A

Chapter 30 Professions and Occupations

Article 7A Practical Nurses

30-7A-1. Definitions

"(a) The term practical nursing means the performance for compensation of selected nursing acts in the care of the ill, injured, or infirm under the direction of a professional nurse or a licensed physician or a licensed dentist, and not requiring the substantial specialized skill, judgment and knowledge required in professional nursing.

(b) The term practical nurse means a person who has met the requirements for licensure as a practical nurse and who engages in practical nursing as hereinabove defined.

(c) The term board as used in this article, shall mean the board of Examiners for LPNS as set forth in section 5 of this article" (West Virginia Legislature, 2016, para. 1)

Table 12.52 Wisconsin

National Council of State Boards of Nursing (2017). Find your nurse practice act: Wisconsin.
Retrieved from https://www.ncsbn.org/npa.htm

Wisconsin Department of Safety and Professional Services (2016). Board of Nursing Licensed,
Chapter N6, Standards of Practice for Registered Nurses and Licensed Practical Nurses.
Retrieved from https://docs.legis.wisconsin.gov/code/admin_code/n/6.pdf

Wisconsin Administrative Code

Wisconsin State Standards 440.08

Chapter N6

Standards of Practice for RN and LPN

N 6.04 Standards of Practice for Licensed Practical Nurses

1) "PERFORMANCE OF ACTS IN BASIC PATIENT SITUATIONS. In the performance of acts in basic patient situations, the L.P.N. shall, under the general supervision of an R.N. or the direction of a provider:

    a) Accept only patient care assignments which the L.P.N. is competent to perform.

    b) Provide basic nursing care.

    c) Record nursing care given and report to the appropriate person changes in the condition of a patient.

    d) Consult with a provider in cases where an L.P.N. knows or should know a delegated act may harm a patient.

    e) Perform the following other acts when applicable:

        1. Assist with the collection of data.

        2. Assist with the development and revision of a nursing care plan.

        3. Reinforce the teaching provided by an R.N. provider and provide basic health care instruction.

        4. Participate with other health team members in meeting basic patient needs.

2) PERFORMANCE OF ACTS IN COMPLEX PATIENT SITUATIONS. In the performance of acts in complex patient situations the L.P.N. shall do all of the following:

    a) Meet standards under sub. (1) under the general supervision of an R.N., physician, podiatrist, dentist or optometrist.

    b) Perform delegated acts beyond basic nursing care under the direct supervision of an R.N. or provider. An L.P.N. shall, upon request of the board, provide documentation of his or her nursing education, training or experience which prepares the L.P.N. to competently perform these assignments.

3) ASSUMPTION OF CHARGE NURSE POSITION IN NURSING HOMES. In assuming the position of charge nurse in a nursing home as defined in s. 50.04 (2) (b), Stats., an L.P.N. shall do all of the following:

    a) Follow written protocols and procedures developed and approved by an R.N.

    b) Manage and direct the nursing care and other activities of L.P.N.s and nursing support personnel under the general supervision of an R.N.

    c) Accept the charge nurse position only if prepared for the responsibilities of charge nurse based upon education, training and experience beyond the practical nurse curriculum. The L.P.N. shall, upon request of the board, provide documentation of the nursing education, training or experience which prepared the L.P.N. to competently assume the position of charge nurse" (Wisconsin Department of Safety and Professional Services, 2016, p. 2)

Table 12.53 Wyoming

National Council of State Boards of Nursing (2017). Find your nurse practice act: Wyoming. Retrieved from https://www.ncsbn.org/npa.htm

State of Wyoming Legislature (2017). Wyoming Statutes, 2016 Constitution, Title 33 Professions and Occupations, Chapter 21 Nurses. Retrieved from https://legisweb.state.wy.us/NXT/gateway.dll?f=templates&fn=default.htm

Wyoming Statutes
2016 Constitution
Title 33 Professions and Occupations
Chapter 21 Nurses
33-21-120 Definitions
Practice of Practical Nursing

"Means the performance of technical services and nursing procedures which require basic knowledge of the biological, physical, behavioral, psychological, and sociological sciences. These skills and services are performed under the direction of a licensed physician or dentist, advanced practice RN, or registered professional nurse. Standardized procedures that lead to predictable outcomes are utilized in the observation and care of the ill, injured, and infirm, in provision of care for maintenance of health, in action directed toward safeguarding life and health, in administration of medications and treatments prescribed by any person authorized by State law to prescribe and in delegation to appropriate assistive personnel as provided by state law and board rules and regulations" (State of Wyoming Legislature, 2017, para. 13)

Printed in the United States
By Bookmasters